Type 1 Di...
Beg...

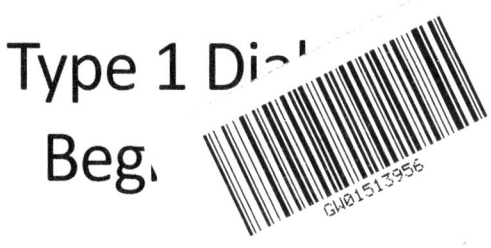

b.

INTRODUCTION

CHAPTER 1 – SO YOU'VE BEEN DIAGNOSED WITH T1 DIABETES

CHAPTER 2 – UNDERSTANDING SUGAR LEVELS

CHAPTER 3 - FOOD

CHAPTER 4 – INSULIN & INJECTIONS

CHAPTER 5 - EXERCISE

CHAPTER 6 - HYPOS

CHAPTER 7 – ALCOHOL

CHAPTER 8 – CHECKING YOUR HEALTH

CHAPTER 9 – PROGRESS IN TECHNOLOGY

CHAPTER 10 – FINDING THE BALANCE

CHAPTER 11 – PERCEPTIONS AND MISCONCEPTIONS

CHAPTER 12 – KNOWING OTHER DIABETICS

CHAPTER 13 – BE YOUR OWN DIABETIC

Introduction

Firstly, thanks for picking up my book. This is my first one. I'm hoping that lots of people read it so I can justify writing another one. We'll see how that goes.

My book is about Type 1 Diabetes. I've been Diabetic since 1995 when I was 14 years old. With a solid twenty-one years under my belt, I now want to share what I think I have learned. My aim whilst writing the book has been to write something that might be useful for newly diagnosed Diabetics – of all ages. I'm hoping parents, friends and family might also find it a worthwhile read.

Whilst in the proofreading stage of writing this book, I sent it to a couple of friends; both of whom I have known for a long time and both of whom I have talked to about my Diabetes. Their reaction to reading my book was a little surprising but was also one that gives me hope that plenty of others could find the book useful. On reading the book, they were taken aback by how little they knew about the condition I have been living with since the day I met them. They were both glad to have read it and feel a little more informed about me since having done so. So if you have any mates you think could do with knowing a little more about you, it could do you good to pass it around.

The book is written in a relatively informal tone. At least that was my intention. There are no charts or tables or any medical jargon. I wanted to avoid all that. What it does contain is real-life advice on how to go about being a Type 1 Diabetic. And, of course, there are a few personal anecdotes included in between.

By no means have I spent the last twenty-one years as a model Diabetic. I do OK. But I am sure I have some decent advice for newcomers to the condition. As a newly diagnosed teenager, I felt there was a lack of real-life guidance out there for me. The doctors would tell me what not to do but I didn't really have much support in figuring out how to continue doing the things I wanted to do. This is the book I would have wanted to read as that teenager.

The book is put together relatively simply. I wanted to cover all the main questions a newly diagnosed Type 1 Diabetic would ask. Hopefully I haven't missed anything too obvious. It is written as a pocket guide to Type 1 Diabetes. I want readers to be able to pick it up and read a chapter now and again rather than just reading it once and putting it in a box to be forgotten. So please feel free to start from wherever you like.

I hope you enjoy the book and are able to take a few nuggets of information away with you.

I would love some feedback from you. Please take a minute to tell me, and others, what you think by leaving a review from wherever you found the book. You can also find me at my blog. Please follow me at

https://t1dbeginnersguide.wordpress.com/

Chapter 1 – So You've Been Diagnosed With Type 1 Diabetes

So you got diagnosed with Type 1 Diabetes. If you are anything like I was when I was diagnosed at the age of 14, you will be going through a mixture of emotions. Life is hard enough – especially when you're a kid. So adding a broken pancreas in to the mix can be a little hard to swallow. But, for whatever reason, this is when Diabetes likes to strike. The majority of Type 1 Diabetics are diagnosed prior to the age of 16.

I remember feeling horrendous in the few weeks leading up to my diagnosis. You probably went through a similar bunch of symptoms as me. You were thirsty all the time. You were making relentless trips to the toilet where you would produce surely more liquid than you had been drinking. And you were constantly exhausted. Even more exhausted than usual. I was 14. I was always tired and always miserable. I used to leave the house at 7.30am for school and walk to the bus stop with my eyes shut just for those extra few moments of near sleep. Then I would sleep for the whole hour on the bus to school before arriving for assembly. And this is before I started to feel ill. The weeks leading up to my ending up in hospital were bad. I was more tired than usual. I would wake up in the morning exhausted having spent most of the night stumbling between my bedroom and the bathroom. I would sleep in lessons. Teachers hated me.

I was a skinny 14-year old but lost even more weight in the weeks prior to diagnosis. I played football and I remember my performances getting worse and worse, being totally drained after five minutes of running about and, more than anything, my teammate's comments about my build. I was literally fading away – and it wasn't as if I had much fat to burn to start with. Where was all this weight going? What was happening to me? I knew something was up. Teenagers can be pretty tactless at the best of times, but the usual teasing felt worse than ever as I could feel something in my body giving up on me. Little did I know at the time that my pancreas had stopped working. Like most 14-year olds, I had never heard of a pancreas.

I remember complaining to my Mum about having a dry mouth all the time. She told me to try mouthwash. I also remember sitting in my living room drinking Lucozade Orange drinks to quell the thirst. In hindsight, not a very good choice of drink. I would be getting up continuously in the night to go to the toilet and remember being scared of the bus trip home from school. I lived eight miles away from school which equated to a one-hour bus trip through various villages. One afternoon we had made it within fifteen minutes of my village before I had to jump off the bus and in to a nearby public toilet. The bus driver wasn't showing much sympathy that day and decided not to wait. I realised at that moment that my whole life had been taken over by the regularity with which I needed to piss. I couldn't even make a one-hour journey on a bus anymore. My teachers were wondering why I needed to go to the toilet mid-way through every lesson. And why I spent the rest of the time asleep.

Something was obviously wrong but I couldn't figure out what it was.

Teenagers are not very good at sharing things. I wasn't. And school is not a place where you get away lightly with showing weakness. Growing up is often a lonely experience and these things happening to you are scary and difficult to figure out. And without understanding all the stuff that's going on, it's impossible to explain it to others. I had a good circle of mates who knew there was something wrong with me and cut me a bit of slack, but none of us at the time were really equipped with the soft skills necessary to talk about it. The lack of a person to talk to as a teenager can make the whole experience a lot worse than it already is.

When you don't know what Diabetes is, you won't ever consider that you have it. I knew all these things were happening but I didn't know why. All I knew was that it was scary and that I didn't really have anyone to confide in. I think that's life as a young teenager. So when my Mum finally took me to the doctors, I felt total relief. Finally someone would take five minutes to explain what was happening to me. Ultimately, it took less than that. The doctor looked at me, I told him my symptoms and he told me I was probably Diabetic. A finger prick to check my sugar level confirmed it. I don't remember the exact number but it was sky high. I was promptly whisked off to hospital. Upon arriving at the local hospital I remember being shoved in to a wheelchair and wheeled down a corridor. At the time I thought this was a bit over the top but it shows how ill I was and also how late I had left it before getting myself to a doctor. But I was actually glad for it. I had been ill for weeks without really doing anything about it. Finally I was in the hands of some people who would look after me.

During my fifteen minutes at the doctor's surgery, I had been filled in very quickly about what Type 1 Diabetes was. I knew it involved having injections. I didn't mind that. I didn't care. If injections were going to fix me and make me feel better then no problem. I can stick needles in myself. So after a blood test and a quick chat, the doctor called the local hospital and instructed them to expect my arrival. My Mum drove me.

My hospital experience was overall pretty pleasurable. The doctors and nurses were initially undecided where to put me. Eventually they decided that I was too old to be put on a kids' ward so I ended up in a bed on a ward surrounded by pensioners suffering with various ailments. I didn't mind. I was being looked after and people were telling me that I would feel better soon. That's all I wanted. I didn't have to worry anymore about bus journeys, about being thirsty all the time or about looking like a skeleton on the football pitch. These people would patch me up and life would go back to normal – or near normal.

I had nurses on tap at my bedside and I was hooked up intravenously to some kind of drip. Looking back, it was obviously an insulin drip. I had to wheel the thing around with me every time I needed the toilet. Every hour, a nurse would show up, prick my finger and put some blood on a strip to check my sugar level. This routine would go on all day and throughout the night. A nurse would come round in the dead of night and give me a quick blood test – sometimes when I was fast asleep. I woke up one night to a pack of nurses pouring sugar in to a glass of milk and throwing it down my neck. It turned out they'd gone a bit over the top on the insulin. I hated and still do hate milk but they had poured it down me before I had a chance to complain. After a few days they had figured out how much insulin my body needed and the drip came out of my arm. I spent the next few days learning how to stick needles in myself and how to accurately squeeze blood on to a small square.

When I got out of hospital a week later, my mates were asking a lot of questions. They were even asking me about how I felt. They were worried about me. Little did they know that the scary part was over for me. As soon as the doctor had told me what was wrong with me, I was liberated. I had something, they knew what it was, and they could make me feel better. That's all I wanted – to feel better. And after a week of being looked after by doting nurses and getting my sugar levels under control, I was feeling better. My mates had even come to visit me in hospital. And so I went home and back to normal life as a teenager. With one big, new difference.

How Am I Supposed to Feel?

You will go through a range of emotions before, during and after your diagnosis. And everyone is different. Some kids get diagnosed not long after birth and grow up knowing no other way of life. Others get it later in life. We are most commonly diagnosed as a child but new cases of Type 1 Diabetes in adults are on the rise.

Prior to being diagnosed, you will feel the usual symptoms of fatigue, thirst and endless urination. You may well be feeling very sad and confused about life. And being diagnosed will trigger a whole new range of new feelings such as relief, trepidation and anxiety. These are all normal feelings in your new situation. The important thing to remember is that the worst bit is over. Everything that is going to happen to your body has already happened. Your pancreas has broken - you are now Diabetic. Now you just have to crack on with dealing with your new situation. Your body isn't going to throw anything else at you. How your body feels from now on will generally be a result of your sugar level, which, armed with your insulin, you now have total control over.

The feeling of control will not come right away, however. Over the next few months, and even years, you will go through a series of stages in terms of how you feel about your Diabetes. And there is no set calendar. This book would be easier to write if there was one.

The Honeymoon Period

To be honest, this may or may not happen to you. Everyone is different and your emotions will take their own path. But it is possible that, after a long period of time feeling absolutely terrible, you have been diagnosed and are feeling brighter. You know what is wrong with you and you have the tools to fix it. You are empowered. Your mates are fascinated with your new condition and you are the centre of attention at school/college/the office. You are beginning to get a handle on your sugar levels and you notice how much better you feel when you get them down to where they should be. You're not feeling ill anymore and you're back in to the swing of things again.

This period of fascination may last from a couple of weeks to a couple of months. You may not experience it at all. Maybe you will jump straight in to the feelings of frustration and rejection. But most new things that we experience in life hold initial periods of interest for us. Over the first few weeks of your new life, you should start to see your sugar levels come down as you become aware of the routine and the rhythm that you need to get yourself in to. Everything in these first few weeks is about your Diabetes and your getting a handle on it. But as time moves on and normal life takes over again, the honeymoon period will come to an end. The attention from friends, parents, nurses and doctors will eventually fade away and you will find yourself alone having to battle with your newly diagnosed condition.

Frustration and Rejection

After a while, you may find yourself getting pretty depressed about your Diabetes. Through no fault of your own, you have been lumbered with an illness – an illness you will have to put up with for the rest of your life. You see all of your friends carrying on their normal lives and slowly forgetting about your condition. Everything becomes complicated. Doing sport, going out with your friends, eating, everything you do becomes all about your sugar level. It never goes away. There are no days off. It begins to dawn on you that, like it or not, you can't do anything without first consulting your sugar level.

This is a challenging period for you. And plenty of people have periods of total rejection not long after being diagnosed. The constant pressure of thinking about your sugar levels, your injections and your meal times becomes too much and you choose to ignore it. Some people long to go back to life before Diabetes and do just that. They stop testing their blood, they stop injecting and they go back to doing what they want. But it doesn't usually last long. A day off the meds and your sugar level will be through the roof. You will soon be reaching for your insulin again. So by all means, have a day off. But you will quickly figure out the result and get back to your new routine. You will slowly discover and begin to accept that, like it or not, you are stuck with this thing. And also that the better you manage it, the better you will feel.

Acceptance and Adaptation

Following a period of struggle, you will at some stage come to a time where managing your Diabetes becomes the norm. You'll forget that there was a time when you didn't have it and will become accustomed to the daily routine of diet, injections and blood testing.

Your Diabetes will forever be a pain in the arse. There is no getting away from that. But you get used to it. You stop fighting with it and accept it as part of your day. Sport, going out with friends, eating out and everything else you want to do is all stuff that you figure out over time. Managing Type 1 Diabetes is one long trial and error experiment. You will never perfect it and you should always be learning from your mistakes. This becomes normality after a while and both life and your sugar level will start to settle down.

What Is This Thing I've Got And Why Did I Get It?

Type 1 Diabetes is an auto-immune condition. Your own immune system has attacked your pancreas, the gland in your body that releases insulin, and rendered it incapable of doing so ever again. The insulin that your pancreas had previously been creating was used by your body to regulate the amount of sugar going in to your blood. Without insulin, sugar piles in to your bloodstream unregulated, causing you the symptoms previously discussed and, if left untreated, also causing a fair bit of damage to your insides. So, without a functioning pancreas, in order to regulate the amount of sugar going in to your blood when you eat, you have to inject insulin in to your body instead.

Let's be honest. Before you were diagnosed with Type 1 Diabetes, you didn't know what it was either. Maybe you heard your mate's Mum has it or maybe even your Granddad or your Uncle has it. But there are two different types and you never really got your head around it. Well, that's the situation your mates are in. That's the situation most of the population are in. They hear things carelessly reported on the news about Diabetes and that eating too much cake will give you Diabetes and that so-and-so is now Diabetic because they're so fat. What the average person gets told about Diabetes leads to a multitude of misinterpretations.

The Diabetes you are used to hearing about on the news is Type 2 Diabetes. This is a different kettle of fish completely. Type 2 Diabetes is not an auto-immune condition. A Type 2's pancreas does still create insulin but not enough to enable it to regulate the sugar in your blood. Some Type 2s are insulin resistant which means the body is unable to use the insulin it creates effectively. Type 2 can also be affected by a poor diet. Or purely by age. This is the one that you hear about on the news being loosely referred to as 'Diabetes.' This is the one your Gran has.

Making a clear distinction between Type 1 Diabetes and Type 2 Diabetes is an important start for you and for anyone you need to explain your new condition to. There is more to come later in the book regarding Type 1 vs Type 2 and the misconceptions that exist around Diabetes.

So, you're not Diabetic because you're too old. You're not Diabetic because you're too fat. Neither are you Diabetic because you ate too many sweets. You are Type 1 Diabetic because your immune system killed the part of the pancreas that is responsible for creating insulin. Scientists are yet to discover why the immune system does what it does. And there are a load of other auto-immune conditions for which we can give no real explanation. Multiple Sclerosis and Arthritis are other examples of auto-immune conditions in which the immune system attacks parts of the body it shouldn't be attacking. Until scientists know any better, getting Type 1 Diabetes or any other auto-immune condition is pure bad luck/fate/whatever you want to call it.

Chapter 2 – Understanding Sugar Levels

What Is My Sugar Level?

OK so your pancreas is broken. It doesn't create insulin. Which means that it won't be regulating your sugar level anymore. That's now down to you. From here on in it's a game. A numbers game. The game is to, in whatever way you can, keep your sugar level as healthy and as steady as possible. It's not about keeping it low. It's not about keeping it high. It's about keeping it steady – or 'within range.'

You will manage your sugar level through a balancing act of diet, exercise and insulin injections. And you will have to monitor your sugar levels to see how good a job you are doing. We do this every day through finger prick blood tests. You prick your finger, drop some blood on to a strip and it tells you how much sugar there is in your blood.

There are two different measurements for our finger prick blood tests. One measurement is mmol/L (millimoles per litre) and the other is mg/dL (milligrams per decilitre). When I was diagnosed in the UK in 1995 everything seemed to be measured in mmol/L. Twenty-one years later and the UK seems to be moving over to measuring in mg/dL which is already standard in Europe and America. My last blood tester was shipped to me by post from Holland and only measures in mg/dL. It has become the internationally preferred measurement for finger prick blood glucose readings. So, from here on in, I will refer to daily blood glucose measurements in mg/dL.

An easy conversion from mmol/L to mg/dL is mmol/L x 18 = mg/dL

So what is mg/dL? Well, mg is a milligram and dL is a decilitre. There are ten decilitres in a litre. So mg/dL basically tells us how many milligrams of sugar are within each decilitre of blood. That's the technical stuff. But all we really need to know is what numbers we should be seeing.

A non-diabetic's blood sugar level throughout the day will be somewhere around 100mg/dL. When that person eats, their pancreas releases insulin and their blood glucose level will remain at or around the same level. The insulin their pancreas releases regulates the amount of sugar in their blood. That is the basic function of the pancreas and the reason why we need insulin. A Type 1 Diabetic's pancreas does not release insulin. So, when we eat, we have to inject what we think is the right amount of insulin for the food we have eaten. The goal is to keep it as close to that 100mg/dL as possible.

However, a Type 1 Diabetic's sugar level will never consistently be as steady or as unswervingly low as that of a non-Diabetic. We inject insulin when we eat but we cannot exactly recreate the job a functioning pancreas naturally does. However well we manage our levels, they will still go up and down more than a non-Diabetic's will. You may well have already read a multitude of information about what your sugar level should be and how you should do everything in your control to keep it steady at 100mg/dL. That's not always realistic. Not if you want to go outside and have a life at the same time. While we are busy living our life, our Diabetes management will have good days and bad days. But while consistently perfect sugar levels aren't always realistic, good management certainly is.

So what is good control? Different doctors and nurses will give you slightly varying top end figures but a good range is between 100-160mg/dL. Trust me – if you are able to keep your glucose levels under 160mg/dL on a daily basis then you are doing great.

In reality, however, your levels will at times go over 160gm/dL. Of course they will. You are not a machine or a walking pancreas. You have a life and you have stuff to do. This is perhaps where my book will vary from the other stuff you have been reading since being diagnosed. I resented most of the things I read about Diabetes after being diagnosed. A lot of what I read gave me the impression that, if I wanted to be a responsible person and look after my health and my glucose levels, I should never leave the house, I should test my sugar level every five minutes and only ever eat what a book told me to eat. Life is not like this. Maybe if I lived like that I would survive until I'm 100. But that's not what being Type 1 Diabetic is all about. It's about leading the life you want to lead whilst managing your sugar levels as best you can. Be on top of it – but be realistic.

Regular Testing

Regular blood sugar level checking is the key to getting a proper handle on your Diabetes. Simply put, Diabetics who check their levels regularly will have better long-term levels than someone who doesn't. Knowing your sugar level also allows you to go about your day freely without having anxieties about your levels in the back of your head all day. And that is the trick to Diabetes. Confidence in our sugar levels and knowledge of what makes them go up and down frees us up to do what we want with our time.

You should check your sugar levels at least four times every day. Without fail you should take a minute before every meal and before bed to check on your levels. The decision you make at meal time on the amount of insulin to inject should be based on both the food you are about to eat as well as what your current sugar level is. And, of course, you can only do this accurately having tested your blood first. You should also get in to a routine of checking your levels before bed. We are asleep for seven to eight hours a day so having a good sugar level for that period is important.

Remember to test your sugar level after eating sometimes too. It's important to test before we eat so we can accurately decipher how many units of insulin we are going to need with our meal. But our blood tests are only snapshots of what is going on across the period of a day. Testing only before meals won't always give you an accurate idea of what is happening to your levels throughout that day and how your levels react to certain foods. Your sugar level will of course increase after eating, but if you can show that your levels are still within range an hour or two after eating then you know you are eating the right foods and are injecting the right doses. I usually have five blood tests each day: one before each meal, one before bed and then an extra one an hour or two after a meal to check I'm not having big spikes in my levels after eating.

Get used to having your blood tests and try to get competitive with yourself on your levels. Set yourself targets and try to improve from week to week.

Trial and Error

Your sugar levels will go up and down. Somehow, injecting manufactured insulin, while it is some amazing science, is not quite the same as having a real pancreas doing it for you. When you eat, your sugar level will go up – even though you will be injecting at the same time. Be aware of this. In the early days after your diagnosis, test your sugar level as often as possible. Get your doctor to put as many test strips on your prescription as possible. This is how you will learn how your glucose level reacts to the different foods you eat.

Make a chart. This might sound over the top – but it's a useful thing to do for a day at least. Pick a day on which you have a normal routine – like a school day or a work day or whatever your routine happens to be. Test your sugar level every hour. Mark down what time you ate, exactly what food you had and how much insulin you took. Then, the next day, sit down and reflect on where your levels went up and down. Did they slip out of range at any stage during the day? How much did they go up after eating? How long did it take for them to begin to come back down again? Why? What did you eat? What if you had eaten potatoes instead of pasta? Try that next time and see what the difference is. Trial and error alongside regular blood testing is how you will quickly start to figure out how food and insulin affect your sugar levels and what the best combinations are to keep your levels within that 100-160mg/dL range.

Make a chart again a week later but eat different foods and try different amounts of insulin. This will help you begin to understand the impact of different foods on your sugar levels. Every time you do this you will learn something. And even if you've been Diabetic for twenty-one years like I have, it's still a smart thing to do. Your body will continue to change throughout your life and you will always be reacting and adapting.

Life as a Type 1 Diabetic is a constant game of Trial and Error. Sitting back and analysing your levels over a day will help you make the adjustments that you need to. If you notice that your sugar level went too high after eating lunch then you have two simple options the next time you eat that meal. Either eat less food or inject more insulin. It sounds simplistic but that really is it. Try the same food but with two more units of insulin next time and see what difference that makes. Or you might figure out that there was something sugary in the meal you ate that you can take out for next time. However you do it, keep testing and keep adjusting.

Testing your blood glucose level regularly is the absolute key to keeping your levels steady. Don't be shy about it. Let people stare. Take your meter absolutely everywhere you go. Check it on the bus, in the pub, at the library, wherever you feel like you need to know. A mistake I made as a newly diagnosed teenager was of somehow being embarrassed about my condition. I would find a toilet to go and have my injection in. I would be too shy to take my blood glucose meter out and about with me and test my levels in front of other people. Please don't make that mistake. Get the people around you used to seeing you testing your sugar level. They will soon understand what you're doing and get bored of staring at you. Or they might even take an active interest and help you out by reminding you to do it. Either way, take your meter everywhere and check your levels regularly.

Make a night time chart too. I always think my blood glucose test before bed is the most important one of the day. Even if I have had a terrible day with my levels, night time is an easy opportunity to get a good level for a seven or eight hour stretch. And your levels are more likely to be good throughout the day if you wake up on a good number. So, record what you ate for your dinner, what time you had it and how much insulin you took. Make a note of your levels before bed and see what it is when you wake up. Depending on your insulin dose and the food you ate for your dinner, you will find that your sugar level does move around while you're asleep. If you ate too late then you might find that your sugar level in the morning is a lot higher than it was before bed. Again, it is trial and error.

Find Your Routine

As a Type 1 Diabetic, routine is your friend. Luckily, most of us have one. Whether you are at school, at college, at university, at work or wherever, most of us do pretty much the same thing for at least five days a week. This is a good thing. For a start, it means we can have breakfast at the same time. And let's be honest, most of us have pretty much the same thing every day for breakfast. So that should be an easy start to the day. You will quickly figure out the right dose of insulin to take with your usual breakfast to see you through until lunchtime.

Try to eat lunch at a similar time each day. Check your levels before your lunch. Learn which meals need which dose of insulin. Add on a bit of extra insulin if your pre-lunch levels are a bit high. This is all the usual trial and error stuff. It will become the norm quite quickly in your day-to-day routine.

I used to play football after work every Monday night. Exercise burns sugar and will reduce your sugar level. After some trial and error, I quickly learned how much extra sugar I would need before playing 7-a-side for an hour. I also sussed out how much extra sugar a 2-mile run would require, or a 90-minute game of football on a Saturday. Most of the things we do in our lives are things we have done before at some stage. So after a while you should know which foods require those extra units of insulin and which activities need some extra sugar.

After being diagnosed, try to get in to your old routine as quickly as you can. If you can start to nail your sugar levels for five days a week then you are doing well.

Diabetes is a diet. So think of it like any other diet. I try to get it right Monday to Friday and then do the best I can at the weekend when I have less of a routine.

Weekends are always more difficult for me; generally because they involve more exercise, more alcohol and less routine. Getting up at different times will also mean different levels and different meal times. A Saturday lay in will mean a later breakfast than usual. Which will in turn mean later lunch and dinner. Eating out means that you are sometimes guessing a little as to exactly how much insulin to take with your meal. Going to the pub or a nightclub on a Saturday night generally involves drinking alcohol. All these things will mess with your sugar levels but are also part of our lives. I don't want to stop doing things I like doing just because I'm Diabetic. I try to fit my Diabetes around it all. So take your blood glucose meter everywhere you go and do the best you can. There are chapters on Food, Exercise and Alcohol later in the book.

Your Blood Testing Kit

The bits and pieces you use to test your sugar level are available at most big chemists/pharmacies you walk in to. With the recent rise in cases of Type 2 Diabetes, more and more manufacturers are releasing blood testing kits. They generally consist of three things. Your meter, the test strips you put in to your meter and the pricker that you prick your finger with. And I am sure you know the process by now. You put the test strip in the meter, prick your finger, drop a tiny amount of blood on the test strip and wait a few seconds for your score. The whole process takes less than a minute. I have to buy my own meter from the pharmacy but I get my test strips on my prescription from the doctor.

Back in the 1990s when I was first diagnosed, I can remember dropping my blood on to a strip and having to wait 30 seconds to see what colour it went. I would then have to compare the colour to those on a chart and try to figure out roughly what my sugar level was. The colours were all shades of yellowy green and it used to take a few discussions before you loosely agreed on what your sugar level might be. So, even in the twenty odd years I have been Diabetic, technology has come a long way. Meters are becoming more and more multi-faceted too. Most these days will give you a detailed history of your last few weeks' test results. Meters nowadays will also give you an average of your levels over the last week or two weeks if you can figure out the right buttons to press. This is all useful stuff. Make sure you set the date and time on your meter correctly so you can track them if you want to.

Along with meters giving you readings and some historical data, you can also use apps to track your levels. There are a few apps available on which you can record your daily test results and track your levels over a longer period. By doing this you might be able to find some times of the day where your sugar levels regularly peak or drop – and be able to adjust your insulin dose or your diet accordingly. This brings me back to the making of a chart. If, either with pen and paper or through something a bit more technologically advanced, you can track your levels over the period of a day or even a week, you will be able to do some good analysis of your levels and quickly suss out reasons behind any highs or lows you might be having.

There are technological advances going on in the management of Diabetes every day. A particular advancement that I am pretty fanatical about is CGM – Continuous Glucose Monitoring. After years of talk, this seems to be starting to come about. And it does exactly what it says on the tin. The technology involves having a small sensor implanted somewhere under the skin with an ability to send blood glucose readings to you every five minutes. Readings can be sent to your phone via an app. I am really excited about this technology. The ability to have 'live' blood glucose readings would be huge for me. I could go about my normal day, briefly glance at my phone every once in a while, as we are all accustomed to doing anyway, and be constantly up-to-date with my sugar level. It would also make it easy to analyse my levels over the period of a day.

Technology really is making it easier for people with Type 1 Diabetes to manage their levels. Take advantage of it. Speak to your doctor, your nurse, your Dietician or whoever you meet regularly. Keep up-to-date on various websites or message boards with what is going on. Figure out what it is you think would make your life easier and go look for it. The chances are someone has already made it or is in the process of doing so. CGM would be an amazing advance for me and I am keeping tabs on it to make sure I can get hold of it whenever it is available to me. There is more on CGM and other new technology in Chapter 9.

Chapter 3 - Food

Understanding Carbohydrates

As a Type 1 Diabetic, you need to understand food. You need to begin to think about and measure the nutritional values of the food you eat. You need to know about carbohydrates, fats, protein and everything else that goes in to the stuff you eat. In particular, you need to start understanding carbohydrates. When you eat, it is the carbohydrates that your body ultimately breaks down and releases in to your blood as sugar. It is the carbohydrate value of the food you eat that will affect your sugar level. So this is what you need to understand in order to inject the correct doses of insulin and to keep your sugar level on the straight and narrow.

We can all name the textbook carbohydrate foods. Bread, pasta, rice, cereal, potatoes. Most people will eat at least one of these foods with every meal - and this is no bad thing. The thing you need to start sussing out is the differing carbohydrate qualities of the foods that you eat and how much of each you should be eating with each meal. Without getting scientific about it, you fundamentally need to know what each of these foods will do to your sugar level in the hours after you have eaten them. Then you can start injecting the correct levels of insulin to match those carbs. And you guessed it, this is a trial and error learning process.

Look on the back of any food packet and you will find the nutritional values of what you are eating. Whether you are eating a bag of crisps, cooking pasta or making a jam sandwich, all the usual nutritional values will be there for you. And you may initially be surprised by which foods have the higher carbohydrate counts. It isn't only the traditional 'starchy' foods that have carbohydrates. Fruits, not traditionally regarded as a carbohydrate based or sugary food, have a lot of natural sugars in them that will go in to that carbohydrate value. A fruit salad may release more sugar in to your blood than a packet of biscuits will.

You should aim to include a low carbohydrate content with each meal you eat. A low carb intake will require a relatively low dose of insulin and will make it a lot easier for you to manage your sugar levels. Larger quantities of carbs make it more difficult for you to keep your levels within range. Big bowls of rice and pasta or foot-long baguettes are generally a bad idea. These big quotas of carbs require equally big doses of insulin and will cause fluctuations in your sugar level. The key to Type 1 Diabetes is to keep a consistent, steady sugar level. You will achieve this best through a low carb diet. The less insulin you are having to inject, the easier it is to keep your levels on a relatively steady plain.

Every meal you eat will have a different mix of foods and different levels of carbohydrates. You will quickly find that your sugar level will behave differently depending on which, as well as how many, carbs you have eaten.

Carb Counting

Different foods have different quantities of carbohydrates. You should get to know how many carbohydrates you are eating with each meal so you can decide accurately how many units of insulin to inject with it. After so many years of being Diabetic, I can quite accurately and instinctively guesstimate what dose of insulin I need with each meal. I have eaten most meals before and I have found the right number of insulin units to go with it. If I wanted to be really accurate, I could even weigh my foods before I cook them just to make sure I am eating consistent quantities. A more scientific and precise method of this guesstimation is called Carb Counting.

Carb Counting involves measuring the grams of carbohydrates in each meal and assigning a number of units of insulin to inject with each gram. A certain weight of each food will have a carbohydrate gram value assigned to it. To count your carbs, you simply total up the number of grams of carbs you are eating for that meal and then inject the assigned number of insulin units. As for the assigned number of units of insulin, everyone is different. You might find you need 1 unit of insulin per 10 grams of carbs. Or you might find that you need 1.6 units – or whatever. This is something you will begin to suss out once you start measuring those carbs you are consuming. Soon you will figure out how much insulin you need per gram of carbohydrates and be able to accurately select the correct dose for each meal.

The information on the number of grams of carbs per food is easy to find. The back of a packet of food will give you all the information you need. You just need to weigh the food before you cook it. Of course, if you buy your fruit and veg at the market, you aren't going to be given a packet with the same information. But no problem. The information you need is easy to find. The internet is full of information on nutrition. There are plenty of websites that you can go to to find all the nutritional information you need. Whatever you eat, it is easy enough to find the carbohydrate values of the food on your plate. There are websites dedicated to Carb Counting that you can use to add up any meal you eat.

There are also stacks of books out there to read on Carb Counting. Take a look at what is available. I use apps. Any app store will have Carb Counting apps available to download – usually for free. A quick scan of a barcode in to your smart phone will often give you all the nutritional information you could wish for. So there is some useful stuff out there. I would advise you to use all the technology you can get your hands on.

It really is as easy as it sounds. The only catch with Carb Counting is having to go through the sometimes arduous task of weighing food and counting up those carbs prior to every meal. Grabbing a quick sandwich becomes a maths lesson all of a sudden. But, of course, in reality you won't have to do this every time you eat. Once you've sussed it out, make a note of how many units of insulin each meal requires and go from there. Grabbing a sandwich at lunch is easy enough to figure out. Just look up the carb value of your two slices of bread, add a little for the other ingredients and you come to your carbohydrate total. Work out the number of units of insulin that total equates to and inject. If you get it wrong then you might have to rethink the number of units of insulin you need for each 10g of carbs. It is trial and error but you will soon get it spot on.

Carb Counting is a great way to educate yourself on the carbohydrate values of the food you eat. But ultimately you won't be doing it for every meal. And counting carbs precisely in a restaurant or café or wherever you choose to eat out is impossible. But a few weeks of Carb Counting and weighing your food will arm you with a much better ability to size up a plate and accurately assess the carb value of what is on there. So do it, go buy a book, get a couple of apps and start counting those carbs. You might not want to do it for every single meal you eat but it's a great way of getting a feel for the carbs in your diet.

The Glycaemic Index

There are different kinds of carbohydrates and each have different release rates. This means that some foods will impact your sugar level almost immediately whereas other slower releasing carbohydrates will impact your sugar level more gradually and over a longer period of time. The rate at which each food will break down in to your bloodstream as sugar is illustrated in something called the Glycaemic Index. The GI classifies foods and gives each one a value. The values range from 0-100. Slow releasing carbs have a low value. Fast releasing carbs have a high value. Glucose itself has a GI value of 100 so gets in to your bloodstream almost as soon as you've swallowed it. This is why glucose tablets are recommended to quickly fix hypos.

White bread has a value close to 90. It is another example of a fast acting carbohydrate that will affect your sugar level quickly. In contrast, wholemeal bread has a value of around 70 so releases sugar in to your blood more slowly and for a longer period of time. This is why it is recommended that you eat wholemeal bread as opposed to white bread at meal times. It is much easier to achieve a steady sugar level by eating foods with lower GI values, drip feeding sugar in to your bloodstream over a period of hours, rather than dumping a load of it straight in there.

So Type 1 Diabetics should eat foods with a low GI value. It helps us keep our sugar levels consistent with no big peaks and troughs. Examples of foods with lower GI values – the foods you should be eating – are: wholemeal bread, pasta, lentils and oats. Porridge is of course made from oats which makes it a much better choice of breakfast than most other cereals.

Higher value GI foods are not necessarily bad for you but they should be avoided in big quantities. Examples of these are: white bread, potatoes and rice. Eating these for dinner will put your sugar level up more quickly than a meal with pasta. It is also important to remember that these high GI foods will not last as long in your bloodstream. They are more likely to put your sugar level up quickly only for it to drop again in a few hours.

Even if you eat the same number of grams of carbohydrates in each, a meal with potatoes will cause your sugar level to react differently compared to a meal including pasta. Let's imagine I have eaten potatoes for dinner and my sugar level is 160mg/dL before bed. Depending on how much insulin and exercise I had with my meal, and how long ago I ate it, I can expect my levels to be back down to near 100mg/dL by morning. However, if I had eaten pasta for my dinner, a lower GI index food and a slower releasing carbohydrate, I would expect to wake up still with a level of around 160mg/dL – if not higher. Pasta will release sugar steadily in to your blood for a few hours. If you have eaten pasta or another slower releasing carbohydrate late in the evening then you might wake up with a higher sugar level than the one you went to bed with.

Testing your sugar level hourly for the four or five hours after a meal will give you a great insight in to the rate at which each food affects your levels. Doing this regularly gives you a great picture of how your sugar level reacts to different carbohydrates in the hours after you eat them. It is a trial and error process. Make charts. Try to learn quickly what foods affect your sugar level in what way. Be conscious of what foods you are eating and how you expect them to affect your levels. Ideally, a low carb diet with low GI values and low doses of insulin will be your best way to keeping your levels consistently under 160mg/dL.

I have really only touched so far here on the foods we traditionally consider to be 'carbohydrate foods.' But remember that most foods have some kind of carbohydrate value and can be found somewhere on the Glycaemic Index. You should include a real variety of food in your new diet. Meat, a small portion of carbs and a big range of vegetables is generally a good option for a meal. Meat actually has a Glycaemic index of 0. It is a protein food that will not have an effect on your sugar level eaten on its own. Vegetables vary but generally have lower GI values, making them a great addition to any plate. Do some studying of the Glycaemic Index and see where your favourite foods are.

Bear in mind that eating lower GI foods with higher GI foods will slow down the rate at which the body absorbs those higher GI foods. For example, a plate of rice will go in to your bloodstream quicker eaten on its own than if you combined it with lower GI vegetables. This makes a healthy mix of food in each meal even more valuable to you.

One other thing to make a note of is that fat slows down the rate of your metabolism. I find takeaway food to release sugar for a really long time. This is why late night takeaways are so bad for my sugar levels. They carry on releasing sugar in to my blood way after I have fallen asleep. Even if you are eating food that you commonly eat, eating it with something fatty can and will reduce the GI value of it. So be aware.

So there is a lot to take in regarding carbohydrates. Take your time learning the different effects of each meal you eat. Enjoying a variety of different foods and avoiding big loads of high GI foods is generally sound advice. Do some reading up on the Glycaemic Index and some experimenting to try and figure out which foods affect your sugar levels in what way.

Of course though, your life as a Diabetic will not be perfection. You will not be the perfect Diabetic. Weighing your food and scanning barcodes for every meal you eat is not realistic. You will eat out, you will wake up late and grab breakfast at the petrol station en route to work. You will eat cake because it's someone's birthday. You will eat takeaway pizza late at night. These things are not found in the Perfect Diabetic textbook but they are of course normal things that you will do in your life. You won't be able to spend all day every day looking at GI indexes and testing your sugar level. But regular blood testing and educating yourself about carbohydrates are important to getting a feel for why your sugar level behaves how it does. Awareness of how foods work and of their carbohydrate values will arm you with the knowledge you need to, as best as you can, match your meals with the correct insulin doses.

Embracing The Food Routine

Like it or not, most of us have a routine. There are loads of different foods in the world – but in reality, we often eat the same meals. Not many of us are gourmet chefs cooking up a range of different dishes each and every night. We regularly eat at home and regularly eat the same kinds of food. As a Type 1 Diabetic, this routine is actually pretty good for us.

It is easy to get daunted by all this info on the GI Index and Carb Counting. Having to figure out all the different properties of food is complex and, for many, not that interesting. But what it boils down to is eating meals and injecting insulin. If you have eaten a meal before, had an injection and your sugar levels were OK afterwards then you can just do the same thing the next time you eat it. That's it.

Try to be consistent with your quantities. Ideally you should weigh your food before cooking it so you know exactly what you are consuming. If that's not realistic then find a different way of doing it. For example, when I eat pasta, I boil a handful of it. That's my measurement and I pretty much know how much insulin that handful is going to require and how my sugar level will behave for the few hours after I eat. I know that because I probably eat pasta 150 times a year. And I've been Type 1 Diabetic for twenty-one years. So what I am saying is this: don't be confused by all the science. If you eat a meal and your sugar level is too high an hour after you eat it, remember to inject more insulin next time you eat the same meal. Or, of course, reduce the quantity you are eating. Very soon you will know exactly how many units of insulin you need for each meal you eat.

If your sugar level is high an hour after eating and has then plummeted within another couple of hours then you should start looking at the GI value of the foods you are eating. If you are having big peaks and troughs in your levels then you should try to head towards lower value GI foods that will help you keep a flatter level by releasing sugars in to your blood more slowly. This makes your life as a Type 1 Diabetic a lot easier. Big peaks and troughs in your levels are not good for your overall Diabetes management. Heading towards lower GI foods and lower insulin doses should keep your levels much steadier.

Meal Planning

Having lived as a single guy for most of my Diabetic life, I have come to appreciate the importance of shopping. I will eat whatever is in the fridge. And, if I can't find anything in the fridge I am likely to get fast-food or a takeaway. So, the food in your fridge will ultimately dictate your sugar levels for the next week or so. Make sure you have in there the things you should be eating.

Ideally you should plan your meals ahead. Whoever does the shopping needs to be pretty strict on what they buy. If you want to eat slow release carbs - low GI foods - then that's what you need to buy. Write a list – plan it – and try not to impulse buy in the supermarket.

We generally eat lunch at work, at college, at school or wherever we spend our day. So, more often than not, we are eating something that can be difficult to put an exact carb value on. But we are still able to make an informed decision about our insulin. Use your experience, count up what's on the plate and try to choose the right dose of insulin. We won't always have access to the scales or to the nutritional information of the food we are eating but the more Carb Counting and GI studying we do, the better informed we are and the better placed we are to suss out the necessary values of any plate of food. Of course, if you want to be in 100% control of what you eat, packed lunches are the way forward. This way you can control exactly what you are eating and be confident in the amount of insulin you are injecting.

As important as *what* you eat can be *when* you eat. Leaving too big a gap between breakfast and lunch can result in your sugar levels dropping before you get to lunch. Again, different GI value foods will affect this. Likewise, squeezing breakfast and lunch too close together can mean that you are eating and injecting for lunch while your breakfast is still breaking down inside you. So be aware. Typically, your sugar level will be higher 3 hours after eating than it is 5 hours after eating. If you are used to testing your sugar levels before lunch then make a note of this. I have made the mistake of over injecting when squeezing meals too close to each other. I have tested my sugar level, seen that it is higher than usual pre-lunch and have over-compensated with extra insulin. But really my levels were quite normal – they were still on their way down after eating breakfast.

This is where making a chart becomes so useful. If you really can accurately assess how your sugar levels react over the course of a day and, importantly, how they curve in the hours after eating a meal, then you will be able to handle eating early or late. In a perfect world, we would leave consistent gaps between meals each day – but that's not always possible. So be aware of the foods you are eating but also of how your sugar levels behave throughout the day. This way you will be better placed to choose the correct dose of insulin and keep those levels steady.

Reacting to Your Sugar Level

We all have weak moments. It might be someone's birthday at school or work or maybe you just fancy pigging out a little on the sofa one evening. Maybe it's Easter and you want an Easter Egg. For all the talk of Carb Counting, weighing food and everything else, you are human and you probably like eating sweet stuff. I do. Maybe you had a rough day and weren't able to keep a hold on your levels. You might have eaten out and got it wrong while trying to count up all the carbs on your plate. Either way, we often get to the end of the day – or even to dinner time – with a higher than expected sugar level.

If your sugar level is high before a meal, inject extra insulin. Some people find a unit of insulin is equivalent to around 20mg/dL. Some will find it is nearer to

30mg/dL. Again, trial and error will help you out here. I generally inject an extra unit of insulin for every 25mg/dL that I am over my usual pre-meal sugar level. But everyone is different so play around with it.

I sometimes get to bedtime with a high sugar level. To be honest, if I have eaten out or been to the pub then this is often the case. In this situation, I have an extra injection before I go to sleep. Night time is an 8-hour opportunity for me to have a good sugar level so I am always keen to take it. Again, I figure that a unit of insulin accounts for around 25mg/dL of sugar. But I am careful to put other things in to the equation too. What did I have for dinner? When did I eat it? When did I have my last injection? How much alcohol did I drink? How much insulin do I really need to take to wake up on a healthy level? You need to be careful with this.

If you are planning on adding an extra injection at any stage during the day, go easy. You don't want to be waking up at 3am suffering from a hypo. This has happened to me – a few times. If you do get to bedtime with a high level and you want to do something about it, start off by injecting 1 or 2 units. Then see how your levels are in the morning. How much did those 1 or 2 units reduce them? Get a handle on how much each unit reduces your levels over night so you can make a more accurate call next time.

Extra injections may not be a textbook Type 1 Diabetes Management technique. You may not find your doctor or many books recommending it. But for me it is a reality. I might have to do it once or twice a week. Ideally you will have perfect sugar levels all day and eat nothing with a GI value of greater than 70. In reality though, you might have eaten out and spent the rest of the night in the pub, or been to McDonalds and got your insulin dose wrong. These aren't things you can get away with doing every day but they are things that you will do from time to time. If you find yourself needing Cheat Injections more than a couple of times a week then you probably need to change your diet or your lifestyle. But just to keep a decent control on your sugar levels in a busy life, they can be useful. But please use cautiously.

Get a Dietician

My ultimate advice on understanding food is this – get a Dietician. Nothing is more valuable than your own experience with food and the lessons you learn through practice. You don't need a Dietician to start Carb Counting or to learn how different GI value carbs will affect your sugar levels. But having someone to bounce ideas off and to introduce you to up-to-date ideas and techniques is great. Everything I have learned about Carb Counting and about the Glycaemic Index began with a conversation with the Dietician.

I find that Dieticians can also be the kick-up-the-backside I regularly need to eat well and look after my sugar levels. Having as many people around me to do this is useful. We can read books, look at websites and follow our own food and insulin regime, but sitting down with someone whose job it is to know about food can be invaluable.

As a summary on food, small quantities of carbs are the best way to go. Low amounts of slow release carbohydrates along with small injections of insulin make it much easier to keep a handle on your sugar levels and keep them consistent. And eat a varied diet. As you get older, you will find that low levels of carbs are a good thing for your body anyway. So be healthy, eat a range of food and get used to counting the carbs on your plate.

Chapter 4 – Insulin & Injections

Injecting

One thing that people will always associate with Type 1 Diabetes is insulin injections. Sometimes it seems to be the only thing that people associate with being Diabetic. This bugs me. People I go out to dinner with will say things like "is that it?" when they see me injecting at the table. Well, no that's not it. The actual act of injecting insulin at meal times is a fraction of what being Diabetic is about. The real work is in the food planning, the testing and the constant consideration we need to give to our sugar levels. I wish it was as easy as just sticking a needle in to myself four times a day. But unfortunately there is a lot more to it.

I got used to injecting myself within a couple of weeks. In reality, it doesn't hurt and the whole thing takes about ten seconds. You will get used to it too. It may take a week or it may take a few months. But eventually it will become second nature and not something you think too much about. At meal times you inject. That's it. As you will have sussed out by now, the real part of being Type 1 Diabetic is figuring out how much insulin you need with each meal and eating the right foods to see your sugar level through to the next meal time.

Technology now offers us alternatives to injecting. In America in particular, insulin pumps are becoming more widespread. In the UK and in Europe they have been slower to appear but they are now doing so. Pumps take away the need for injections but still follow the same theory as injecting with pens. When we eat, we take insulin. Whether you use a pump or a pen to do this, you will still be choosing an insulin dose to take with every meal you eat. You still need to plan the food you eat, your meal times, your exercise and everything else. You still need to consider your sugar levels in everything you do.

Whether you choose to use a pen or a pump to give yourself insulin, it's great to see technology evolving to help out Type 1 Diabetics. And there is more to come, I am sure. There is more on pumps, the advancement of technology and its usefulness in Chapter 9.

What is Insulin And How Often Should I Inject It?

The art of being Type 1 Diabetic is trying to replicate what your broken pancreas was doing before it gave up on releasing insulin. What your pancreas had been doing prior to its meltdown was pretty incredible; as are most of the natural functions of the human body. It produced insulin and got it in to your bloodstream where it regulated your body's sugar level.

Your pancreas doesn't work anymore. That's what being Type 1 Diabetic is. Well, the bit that produces insulin doesn't work anymore. So, you need to manually put insulin in to your body to, as closely as possible, replicate what a functioning pancreas would be doing. This is how I describe Type 1 Diabetes to my friends. I have to do manually what a functioning pancreas does automatically. The closer to the job of a functioning pancreas I can do, the better my sugar levels will be and the healthier I will be.

When I was first diagnosed at the age of 14, I began my new life as a Diabetic on two injections a day. I did this because it was what the doctors at the hospital told me to do. The Diabetic Nurse I saw at a later stage told me nothing different. No other options were discussed. I wasn't told about alternative regimes. So I injected the same insulin twice a day. The insulin was a mixture of basal and bolus insulin inside a single cartridge. I injected at breakfast and at dinner. Looking back on this, it was a terrible idea and I'm not sure why it was ever suggested.

My blunt advice to you is this: have four injections a day – not two. Your life will be simpler, you will have greater freedom over meal times and your sugar levels will be a lot better for it. It wasn't until I was 22 and out of university that I began to inject four times a day. And it was only then that I really began to get a hold of my sugar levels. So don't make the same mistake as me. Have four injections from the start. The more injections you have, the easier your life will be and the easier you will find it is to manage your sugar levels.

So why was I told to have two injections a day? I can only think it was because doctors and nurses at the time believed it was easier for a teenager to deal with two injections a day rather than four. But, as I've said, the injections are something you get used to pretty quickly. They quickly become not a big deal. What I was more concerned about when I was diagnosed, and still am today, was the stress of managing my sugar levels. And two injections a day wasn't good for this. I would have one with my breakfast at 7am before heading off to school. This mixture of bolus and basal was somehow designed for the bolus to peak again around lunchtime. However, I found this happening at around 10am rather than at 12pm when I was actually eating my lunch. By the time I had my lunch, the insulin seemed to have already worn off and I spent the afternoon with high sugar levels. If I had known at the time about the alternative of injecting a bolus insulin with each meal, I would have jumped at the chance of switching regimes.

I remember doing my GCSE exams with a pack of sweets on my table worrying more about my sugar level than about answering the questions. I found that the two injections a day regime ruled me more than I ruled it. It stressed me out. My advice to you is this: if there is anything you can do in your daily regime to reduce stressing about your levels, then do it. Checking sugar levels regularly will help reduce any anxiety about your levels. And so will moving to a multi-injection regime that gives you much more freedom to eat when you want and do what you want without having your insulin regime mastering you.

Your four injections a day should include three bolus injections at meal times as well as one daily injection of basal insulin.

Basal Insulin

Basal Insulin is a long-acting, or 'background' insulin. It is designed to gradually release throughout the periods of the day when we're not eating. Even when we are not eating, our body releases glucose in to our blood to give us energy. Basal insulin helps regulate our sugar level during those times. You should inject a single dose of basal insulin per day.

The basal insulin we inject is manufactured to release inside your body slowly over a period of 24 hours – thus replicating the job of a functioning pancreas. I think of it as a drip-feed insulin quietly doing its job while you go about your daily business. It should be injected at the same time every day – every 24 hours - to keep a constant drip feed of it in to your bloodstream.

You will need to choose a time of day that you are going to do this. Popular times are breakfast time, dinner time or bed time. But choose a time when it is realistic for you to inject at the same time each day. If you get up at 6am for work every day and inject your basal then, ideally you should be injecting your basal at the same time on Saturday and Sunday. If you leave it until 10am one day, you may find your body has run clean out of basal insulin and your sugar levels have already increased by the time you get around to injecting. So make it easy for yourself – pick a time that suits you 7 days a week. I choose to inject my basal at around 7pm each day. I am generally home from work then and it is also an easy time to choose for weekends or any time I am out of my usual routine.

You may find that your basal insulin doesn't last for a whole 24 hours. Although it is designed to work for an entire day, it may actually only last for 20 hours or so. I find that eating after 2pm has a bigger effect on my sugar level than eating at any other time. I think this is because the basal insulin I injected the previous evening has already begun to run out by then. Every Diabetic is different and there are no absolute rules. You will need to monitor this.

Try to figure out if you are having any strange spikes in your levels that could be explained by a shortcoming in the duration of your basal. Play around with the times you are injecting it at to see what best suits your routine. Some people have experimented by splitting their basal dose in to 2x injections per day – one every 12 hours. If you think you have an issue, experiment with the number of units you take, try splitting it or even try going to your doctor and trying a different brand of basal insulin. Trial and error with your basal insulin will help you understand how it works and ultimately land you on the best regime for you and your lifestyle.

As for the amount of basal you should be injecting per day, this usually mirrors, more or less, your total daily bolus dose. At least that is what you should start on. And it will be what the doctors suggest. But from that starting point, you should play around with it. Get used to trialling different basal doses and measuring the effects.

Bolus Insulin

Bolus insulin is short-acting insulin. It is the insulin we inject at mealtimes to deal with the carbs we put in to our body whenever we eat. A functioning pancreas will automatically release the perfect amount of insulin each time we eat to regulate the sugar level. We have to decide ourselves how much bolus we need for each meal we eat.

Your bolus injections are relatively straightforward. You need to inject one bolus dose with each meal you eat. This is typically three a day: breakfast, lunch and dinner. But if you have four meals a day, you have four bolus injections. Simple. Your bolus insulin is the insulin your body needs to regulate the sugar you are putting in to it whenever you eat food. So figure out how much you need to take for the meal and inject.

In my days as a Diabetic, I have been told different things about exactly when I should have my bolus injection. Twenty years ago I was told that I should have it 20 minutes before my meal to allow for the time it takes to have an effect. But that's not the case anymore. With modern day manufactured bolus insulin, we are advised to inject immediately before we eat. I generally wait until the plate is on the table, do some quick adding up of the carbs I can see, inject and then eat. Of course, before every meal I will check my sugar level first. You can't accurately decide how much bolus insulin to inject without knowing your current sugar level.

Bolus is short-acting insulin. It is designed to deal with the sugar you are eating with each meal. So you need to figure out how much that is and inject the necessary amount of bolus. My tip is, the less bolus you are having to inject, the steadier your levels will be. I am not suggesting you should have less than you require here. I am suggesting that you should generally eat those healthy foods that only require a low amount of bolus. If you find yourself having large bolus doses each meal time then you will probably find you have some pretty spiky sugar levels – with big highs after eating. If this is the case, you will need to find those lower carbohydrate, lower Glycaemic Index foods that can be managed with lower bolus doses and help you maintain steadier sugar levels.

Your bolus dose for each meal should be dictated by some Carb Counting and also by some past experience. Whatever it is that you're having for dinner this evening, you've more than likely eaten it before. So make notes of your bolus dose for each meal you eat and go from there next time you have it. Notes from previous meals alongside some carb counting should soon land you on the right number.

Where Should I Inject?

You should spread your injection sites around your body. I have four injections a day (plus an occasional cheat injection before bed if necessary). So I have four injection sites. I use both of my thighs and the sides of my belly. The thighs seem to take it better than the belly. You will come to understand which parts of your body take to injections better than others. Anywhere with a bit of fat is usually a good choice. As a newly-diagnosed, skinny teenager this was easier said than done;

especially having lost even more weight prior to being diagnosed. But I found a chunk of fat on each thigh and started there. As I got older more chunks appeared and the side of my belly has become a convenient place to stick it whilst sat at the dinner table or out at a restaurant.

Be careful with the areas you inject. Look out for lumps around injection sites. These lumps can be a build-up of fat and scar tissue caused by overuse of a particular area for injections. They are not a serious problem but you should avoid the area for injections until they go away. Insulin can get trapped in these lumps in overused areas and fail to circulate itself in to your bloodstream where it needs to be in order to be effective.

The best advice on injection sites is to spread them around your body as much as possible in order to avoid overusing specific areas. An injection anywhere under the skin will do the job and quickly get in to the bloodstream. So vary it as much as possible and, if necessary, be creative.

I sometimes have a small lump under the skin on my thigh after I inject my basal insulin. This is a big injection compared to the smaller and more regular bolus ones – around 44 units in one go for me. If I notice a lump under the skin immediately after injecting, I give it a rub to make sure the insulin isn't sticking there for too long and within 30 minutes it has usually disappeared. This seems to happen now and again with my big injections but I make sure I spread it up and down my thighs to avoid the appearance of any longer-terms lumps. If you are getting lumps that stay around all day, it is time to avoid that area for a while.

Needles

To fit your pen you can get 5mm or 8mm needles. I have recently gone down from 8mm to 5mm. It seems to be that the shorter needles do less damage to the skin. And if we are asked how long a needle we want to stick in our leg, I think most of us would choose the shorter one.

Make sure you change your needles regularly. It has been recommended to me by a doctor that I should change my needle before every injection. You can do this if you want, of course. But it does seem a little over-the-top to me. I change the needle every 2-3 injections. I keep an eye on my injection sites and they seem to be OK. Leaving it too long between needle changes will result in blunt and damaged needles. So be sensible with your needles, look after your injection sites and make sure you move them around as much as possible.

You should also be careful to dispose of your needles safely when you've finished using them. Your doctor should give you the right equipment for you to do this. Mine end up in a yellow box that I take to a collection point once a month when it's full up. Don't just chuck your used needles in the bin. Your rubbish goes through a multitude of hands once it's been collected and none of them want to get pricked with your old needles.

Your Pens

If you are injecting your insulin then you will be the proud owner of insulin pens. Years ago, Diabetics had to carry around and inject with syringes. Pens are much friendlier looking things. These are what you will, along with your blood tester, need to remember to take with you wherever you go. Take your pens everywhere. You never know when your next meal plans may change. It's also a handy tip to make sure you have enough insulin in them before leaving the house. I have lost count of the number of times I have gone out to eat dinner, taken my trusty pen with me only to realise, just as my food is put in front of me, that the cartridge inside it is empty. So check before you leave the house that your pen has enough insulin in it to see you through the day.

There are two different kinds of pen. One is pre-filled and to be thrown away after use. My basal pen is like this. I use it for a week and once the insulin has run out, it goes in the bin (minus the needle of course). The other kind of pen is a refillable pen. I have used the same refillable pen for my bolus injections for years and years. These refillable pens take cartridges of insulin that you will pick up on your prescription. You stick the cartridge in to the pen, use it until it runs out, chuck the old cartridge away and put a new one in.

Before you have your first injection of a new cartridge, you should check everything is in place properly first. Squeeze out 3-4 units until insulin starts squirting out. Then you are good to go. This avoids injecting fresh air on your first injection of a new cartridge.

If you do have a refillable pen, make sure it is not your only one. Depending on how good you are at losing things, you should have at least one spare. During a night out a few years ago, I managed to lose the only pen I had with me. I think it slipped out of my pocket in a late night taxi. When I woke up the next morning, I was 100 miles from home, hungover and devoid of insulin. Needless to say, it was a long and hungry journey home. So learn from my mistakes and make sure you have spares of everything everywhere you go.

You also need to keep your insulin cool. Your spare packs of insulin should live in the fridge. Ideally your pen should also be in there if you are at home. If you are out and about then just keep it as cool as possible. This is easier in some countries than others. I grew up in England so keeping my pen cool when I was out wasn't too much of an issue. However, in warmer climates you need to think about how you are going to keep your insulin cool. If you are going on holiday, get some kind of insulated pack in to which you can put your pen and keep it at a reasonable temperature.

Be Grateful

It is worthwhile to take a minute to appreciate the rate of advances Diabetes has been through during the last century. A hundred years ago, prior to the discovery of insulin in the early 1920s, Type 1 Diabetes was an untreatable condition. If you got it, you died – quickly. Once insulin was discovered, we began by using insulin from the pancreases of dogs, cows and pigs to treat human Diabetics. That was the beginning of insulin injections. Since then insulin has become mass manufactured and is used to treat Diabetics all over the world. Less than a century after the discovery of insulin, we are continuing to further technology to improve the lives of thousands.

I am from the UK and am lucky to have a National Healthcare that pays for my insulin. In America and plenty of other developed countries this is not the case. Unfortunately people's management of their sugar levels is often dependant on how much money they have in the bank. And a disconcerting number of poorer countries even struggle to afford insulin at all. For many kids around the world, Type 1 Diabetes is still a death sentence. So we with insulin in the fridge have a lot of reasons to be thankful. I hope that, while we continue to advance technology for the privileged, we can work as hard on getting basic insulin supplies out to everyone in the world who needs it.

Chapter 5 - Exercise

Be Healthy

Exercise is a vital part of anyone's life and it should be no different for a Type 1 Diabetic. In the haze of carbohydrates, blood tests and injections, it's easy to overlook the bigger picture. But we need to remember that our health is about more than just our sugar levels. Our general health is important too. Our sugar levels will tell us about our Diabetes management. But, while our management of our levels is and always will be the backbone of our keeping healthy, we shouldn't ignore the other stuff while we're at it.

If I sat in my house doing nothing day after day then I imagine looking after my sugar levels would be easier than it is now. But sitting around doing nothing with our lives doesn't lead to a fulfilling or healthy lifestyle – or a healthy body. Exercise is great for us in a few different ways. It burns fat, builds our muscle and is one of the best natural releases of endorphins you will find. So we need to get out there and exercise – no excuses. We can be healthy and try to manage our sugar levels while we're doing it.

The secret to being Diabetic is to find a way of fitting your Diabetes in to everything you do in your life. Not the other way around. Exercise is no exception. As a kid, I was always sporty. I played a lot of football and continued to after my diagnosis at the age of 14. I sussed out the impact of a football match on my sugar levels and quickly discovered that good sugar level management often resulted in a good performance. Now in my mid-thirties I'm still playing and still battling away with keeping my sugar levels half decent whilst I'm doing it. Managing your sugar levels whilst exercising is not easy – but it is a challenge we should all embrace.

When people find out that I'm Diabetic, they start asking me questions. "Can you do this? How about doing that and that?" The answer to all these "can you" questions is Yes. Yes, I can play football. I can swim, play tennis, go running. I can climb mountains and jump out of planes if I really want to. I can travel around the world. I can do anything I want to. I just have to fit my Diabetes around it the best I can. Exercise is the same. You just need to go out and do it. You may initially find that your sugar levels are difficult to keep a handle on. In fact, you will find that for as long as you live and for as long as you exercise. You may even experience a few hypos here and there. But exercise is great for us and being Diabetic is not an excuse to stop doing it.

How Will Exercise Affect My Sugar Levels?

The first thing you need to know, and probably already know, is that exercise lowers your sugar level. So, when you exercise, you need to do one of two things – or a combination of the two. You need to inject less insulin before exercising and/or you need to consume extra sugar before and during your exercise. For example, I know that I need to reduce my lunchtime insulin dose by half if I am playing a football match that afternoon. I will also need to check my sugar level before the game, at half-time and again at full-time to make sure they are somewhere near where they should be before, during and after my exercise.

Your levels will never be perfect when competing in sport or exercising. Before a football match, I prefer them to be a little higher than usual to avoid any untimely hypos out on the pitch. When I say 'a little higher,' I generally aim for levels of around 180mg/dL at kick-off. I take sugary drinks with me and top up when my sugar levels are dropping below that desired level. Through trial and error, you will find the level you want to be at when exercising. And it can be different depending on the sport you are playing or the exercise you are doing. Football is pretty strenuous and I know that I am out there for 45 minutes at a time. Running marathons, running sprints, playing tennis, playing golf will all impact your sugar levels in different ways and will all have different rules for the amount of extra sugar you want to be taking on.

As well as playing football, I have always played golf and I am always surprised at how much a round of golf drains my sugar levels. Swinging a club and strolling around in the woods for a few hours doesn't sound too strenuous, but walking is exercise too. So you need to carefully consider what actually constitutes exercising. Even taking the dog for a walk will impact your sugar levels and might be as good an excuse as any for a bit of chocolate pre-walk. As a Diabetic, the more exercise you do, the closer you will get each time to figuring out what the right insulin dose or pre-match snack is.

There are various high GI foods that you can take with you when you exercise for fast-releasing bursts of sugar. Glucose itself is of course the fastest acting and there are plenty of glucose tablets out there that you can take with you. I pack these for football matches and find my sugar levels begin to increase within fifteen minutes of eating them. This means that a low sugar level caught at half-time can just about be reversed in time for the second half. There is also a range of sport drinks to take on when exercising. What I would suggest with these is that you read the label carefully. Some of these are based more on caffeine than on actual sugar content. Figure out what is the best food or drink for you and make sure you have enough of it with you whenever you play.

I find that reducing my insulin dose is actually a better way of managing my sugar levels than eating or drinking extra sugar. Taking on extra sugar can be necessary when we exercise but the combination of insulin + sport + sugar can lead to big peaks and troughs in your levels. Bolus insulin is somehow extra-activated by exercise. Through experience, I have found that injecting bolus anywhere within a couple of hours of playing football can often result in a hypo out on the pitch. It's a dangerous combination taken too closely together. Somehow exercise enhances insulin activation and together they drop my sugar level rapidly. However, if I eat at least two hours before I play and have a reduced dose of insulin then I find that there will be fewer unexpected drops in my levels when I am playing. My sugar levels are steadier and I don't need to keep taking on extra sugar.

You need to find your own combination of extra sugar and reduced insulin to suit the exercise you are doing.

As ever, trial and error and regular blood testing is the key.

What Should I Eat Before Exercise?

We are up to Chapter 5 already here so I am hoping you already know the answer to this one. The answer is of course low GI foods. If you can eat a meal that is still releasing sugar in to your bloodstream whilst you exercise then that is ideal for your sugar levels – as well as your energy levels. Before a football match, I eat a big plate of pasta with a load of vegetables. Wholewheat pasta if I can find it. This is a slow release meal that will still be trickling in to my blood as the game is kicking off.

So think about your pre-exercise regime. What time will you eat? What food will you eat? How much are you going to reduce your insulin dose? What sugar level do you want to be on when you begin your exercise? What extra sugar are you going to take with you? This is all stuff you will work out over time. But I have found that it's a difficult one to completely master. Every football match is different, every day is different and my sugar levels are never exactly the same. But I do the best I can. I fit my Diabetes in to my sport – not the other way around.

There are plenty of real-life Type 1 Diabetic professional athletes out there who us amateurs can learn a lot from. Since I was diagnosed, I have followed the progress of Scott Verplank – the professional golfer from America. I have watched Verplank play in two Ryder Cups with his insulin pump attached. Wasim Akram (Cricket) and

Steve Redgrave (multi-Olympic gold medal winning Rower) are two other examples of world class Type 1 Diabetic sportspeople. Novo Nordisk themselves have a cycling team made exclusively from Diabetic cyclists. So we certainly have no excuse for sitting on our backsides. Look these people up and see if you can get some tips from the people who do it for a living.

What Happens After I Exercise?

Keeping track of your levels before and during exercise is important. I have found that equally as important is looking after them once the exercise has finished. On quite a few Saturday nights, my sugar levels have tumbled – even a few hours after finishing my exercise. My body seems to work as hard in its recovery as it does when it's actually doing the exercise. So be conscious of this. Of course, every Diabetic is different, but your levels may still be affected for a good few hours after you complete your exercise.

The best thing to do after exercising is of course to eat. Your body needs to refuel. So get some food in you and help it recover. This is true whether or not you are Diabetic. But be careful with your insulin dose. Remember that your body will still be burning up sugar a little quicker than usual.

Trial and error is the key. Along with regular blood tests. Does this sound familiar? Of course it does. It is pretty much the advice for every aspect of being Type 1 Diabetic. More testing and more trialling will help you understand the impact of exercise on your sugar level.

Testing before, during and after will allow you to see the pattern of the effect on your levels. Try different pre-exercise meals and try different reductions of your insulin dose. You will soon come to figure out the best way to manage your sugar levels whilst doing the things you love to do.

Make Sure People Know

Make sure people know you are Type 1 Diabetic. If you are exercising with friends or playing a team sport this should be easy. Try not to be shy about it. Get your blood tester out and let people ask questions. Try to explain the balancing act involved in managing your sugar levels whilst playing sport. I have always been a little too shy about my Diabetes. It's not natural for me to start telling people about myself. But I find that if I go through my usual routine of blood testing and getting the necessary pre-match sugars on-board, people will quickly enough figure out why I'm doing it and will be asking me questions about it.

People knowing about your Diabetes is crucial for any hypo you might have whilst exercising. When playing football, I can usually feel the symptoms of a hypo coming on and quickly fix it by someone chucking me a sugary drink from the sidelines. In a more serious issue when a hypo strikes a little quicker, it is important for your mates to know that you're having a hypo and that you need sugar. For those who don't understand the ins and outs of Type 1 Diabetes, all they need to know is that. If I am playing sport and I start to look ill, give me some sugar.

Exercising alone is different. There may be nobody around to recognise the signs of a hypo. If you are out running, for example, make sure you have an emergency stash of sugar – and ideally have your blood tester with you. If exercising on your own is a regular thing, you might want to think about some kind of identification to point out to strangers that you are Type 1 Diabetic. In an emergency, a piece of jewellery can quickly advise a helpful bystander that you are Diabetic, you look ill because you are having a hypo and that you need sugar fast.

Managing Expectations

Exercise is an important part of anyone's life. Or it at least should be. Managing your sugar levels whilst doing sport can be quite complex. So I think we really need to cut our expectations to suit. Your levels may not be perfect when you are exercising. You will probably even purposefully, as I do, keep your levels a little higher than usual while doing it. That's OK as long as you can quickly enough sort them out and get them back to normal afterwards. This is life. As we fit our Diabetes around the things we love to do, we have to accept that it's not always possible to have ideal levels. Do the best you can and continue to learn every time you exercise. Trial different regimes of insulin doses and pre-exercise meals. Find out what works best for you.

Remember that exercise will lower your sugar level. So think about what exercise is. I used to have a job that involved sitting in a chair in an office for 8 hours a day.

When I moved on to a job that required me to be on my feet for most of the day, I found that I needed a lot less insulin with my meals. I was burning up sugar much quicker than if I had been sitting in a chair all day. Seemingly small changes to your daily routine can actually have big effects on your sugar levels.

Exercise can take many different forms and all will need a different preparation with regards to food and insulin. The main thing I have come to realise, especially when walking or playing golf, is the importance of a good meal before exercise. If you can get a load of slow-releasing carbs in you before you go out to exercise then you are doing yourself a big favour. Alongside a smaller bolus injection, these carbs should continue to release in to your bloodstream as you exercise, negating the chances of any serious hypos. You will need fewer, or even none at all, sugar top ups as you exercise. So next time you go out to exercise or to play sport, give yourself a big pre-match low GI meal and go from there.

Chapter 6 - Hypos

What Is A Hypo?

'Hypo' is short for Hypoglycaemia and is the term we use for a low blood sugar level. Hypos are unfortunately part and parcel of being a Type 1 Diabetic. But don't fret - they are nothing to be scared of. Hypos can actually be seen as a sign that you are doing pretty well in controlling your sugar levels. It doesn't take too much for your levels to slip underneath where they are meant to be. In fact, Diabetics who have absolutely no hypos are probably spending too much time with seriously high sugar levels. As a Diabetic, hypos need to be accepted as part of life. They will happen. Learn how to detect them early on and they won't cause you too much bother.

The science behind a hypo is pretty simple. They happen when we have too much insulin and not enough sugar in our blood. So we have injected too much insulin for the amount of carbs we had for our last meal. Or we may have over-exerted ourselves during exercise and burnt up all the sugar we had in there. Either way – Hypoglycaemia is a simple case of not having enough sugar in our blood. Non-Diabetics won't suffer from hypos. Their body will only produce an amount of insulin suitable for the amount of sugar they have eaten. We Diabetics, on the other hand, sometimes get our insulin vs food balance wrong and our sugar level will slip a little low.

Your sugar level should be somewhere around 100-160mg/dL. A non-Diabetic's levels will consistently be around 100mg/dL. Hypo symptoms will start to be felt from around 70mg/dL downwards. But don't worry - your body is smart. When your sugar levels begin to drop to around the 70mg/dL mark, it will start to give you some signals that will make it clear to you that you need to eat – and eat quickly.

The lower your blood sugar drops, the more noticeable your symptoms will be. At around 70mg/dL you will begin to feel a hypo setting in. There is no rule about what sugar level you need to get to before you start to feel a hypo – but 70mg/dL is about the level where I notice it. Others may start to feel it a little sooner or even later. The quicker you deal with it the better. Hypos are usually very simple to detect and to manage. However, if left untreated, a hypo can get serious. By the time your levels slip to 30mg/dL or below then you may be struggling to function. By 20mg/dL you will be losing, or will have already lost consciousness.

Serious hypos are rare. I have been Type 1 Diabetic for twenty-one years and have never been hospitalised from a hypo. I think the lowest I remember recording was around 32/mg/dL. Luckily I was still functioning well enough to fix myself with a boat-load of glucose tablets. Being able to recognise the symptoms and always having a source of sugar close to hand should save you from any serious hypos too.

What Are The Hypo Symptoms?

Recognising the symptoms of a hypo is important. The quicker you notice the signs, the more quickly and easily you can deal with it. If I am at work, I will have a bottle of a sugary drink in my bag wherever I go. If I am out and about then I will always have some glucose tablets in my pocket. I deal with most of my hypos very quickly because I can recognise the symptoms. People I am with often don't even know it happened. I will neck half a bottle of juice, try to have a little sit down for fifteen minutes and then carry on with whatever I was doing. Glucose tablets and sugary drinks act very quickly so within that fifteen minute period, sugar levels can return to normal.

There are some very common symptoms that your body will demonstrate to you whenever your sugar level is dropping too low. You may not experience all of those I list but I am sure there will be a few that you will come to recognise. After a few hypos, you will come to understand your own body's way of letting you know that your levels are too low.

Hunger - this is the one my body throws at me first. Even if I have eaten recently, my body will make it really clear to me that I need to eat again – and something sugary. If I wake up in the night and the first thing I notice is hunger, I know what's going on.

Dizziness/Weakness/Shakiness – whatever you want to call it, it is a sure-fire sign of an onsetting hypo. This can be confusing for me on the football pitch. There have been plenty of occasions I have mistaken fatigue for a low sugar level. It is easily done. So if you are ever unsure, get the blood tester out and check.

Blurred Vision – if you are at home relaxing on the sofa, it may be more difficult to notice signs of shakiness. But if you are reading a book or watching TV and your sugar level begins to slip then it may be your vision that you notice going first. A little test I give myself if I am starting to feel a little wobbly is to get my phone out and see if my text messages are looking blurry. If they are then it's usually a sign that I need to get some sugar in me.

Sweating – this is the one that my body saves for a really low level. It is the sweating that most people associate with a hypo and the thing that people you are with will notice. There have been times when my sugar level has dipped under the 50mg/dL mark and I have been drenched in sweat. I remember a time at work when I ended up sitting in front of a fan for half an hour munching sweets with my work shirt totally sodden. It's not a good look. But that was my own fault. I had been sitting in a meeting with no backup sugar on me when I started to notice the signs of a hypo coming on. Rather than bolting out of the meeting, I decided to ride it out until the end. Needless to say, the meeting went on for longer than expected and I ended up with a drastically low sugar level. The lesson from that was an easy one – always have a sugar backup and don't be shy about your Diabetes. If you really need to – go get some sugar.

Numb Tongue – I think this is more of a rare one – but it is something I suffer from during a hypo. For other people it can be a general feeling of pins and needles around their lips and mouth. For some reason my body reacts by giving me a numb tongue. I am not complaining. Any sign my body wants to give me to remind me to go and eat is a useful one.

You will have your own list of symptoms too I am sure. Some might be on my list, some might not be. The important thing to remember is to not be scared of having a hypo. I probably get the symptoms a couple of times a week. I have come to recognise them quickly and it is easy for me to deal with it. And you will only come to recognise your own hypo symptoms by actually having a hypo. They will happen. It is a part of being Diabetic and something you need to learn to deal with as simply and as quickly as possible. Remember that hypos are often a sign of good management. High sugar levels are bad and can cause serious long-term complications. Low sugar levels are a mere temporary inconvenience. Or at least they will be if you become adept at noticing the warning signs and always have that stash of sugar with you.

Over the years, my body has become well-trained at warning me of a low sugar level. Or sometimes even of an impending low sugar level. I am usually a great sleeper. I am asleep as soon as my head touches the pillow. So when this doesn't happen, I know something is wrong. I sometimes go to bed and start to feel hungry. I feel mild signs of a hypo – as if my body is warning me not to nod off. I check my levels and I find them to be around 110mg/dL – definitely not in hypo range. But this is my body's way of warning me that they are on their way down and that I should have a snack before I go to sleep. I can't explain the science behind this. But it happens. My body somehow knows when to give me those symptoms. So, listen to your body. Generally you will find that if you need to eat, your body will let you know one way or another.

What Do I Do If I Have A Hypo?

This might seem like a silly question. Of course, if your sugar level is low then you need to eat sugar. Or drink sugar. It's that simple. But it can be more complicated than just getting your glucose tablets out. Ideally you will recognise the symptoms quickly and be able to deal with it with a quick bite or drink of something sugary. But if you are slow to notice the onset then you might be relying on others to help you out. This is why I always make the point of making sure that the people around you know about your condition. And, in a worst case scenario, make sure strangers can tell by carrying some clues on you.

If your levels drop seriously low (maybe sub 35mg/dL) you may become somewhat unaware of what's going on. If it continues to drop then it's likely that you will fall unconscious. Totally untreated hypos can lead to a coma. But, if you carry sugar with you wherever you go then you should be able to avoid anything this serious.

Those around you need to know what to do in a situation where you are unable to give yourself the necessary sugar. If they are able to then they should get a sugary drink inside you quickly. Even in a semi-conscious state, most of us can still swallow liquids. If you are incapable of swallowing then rubbing sugar in to your gums will do the trick. Of course, if you are past the point of being able to feed yourself then you will need a lot of sugar. Rubbing sugar in to your gums should get you to a point where you are back with it and able to swallow something again. The sugar will take 15 minutes to get in to your bloodstream and for you to be showing signs of recovery.

The point to make here is that prevention is always better than the cure. Carry sugar with you and make sure people around you know that you are Diabetic as well as what they need to do in an emergency.

Your Backup Sugar Stash

OK so you have probably got the point by now. But wherever you go, make sure sugar is close to hand. It will give you the freedom to go about your daily life without having to worry too much about impending hypos. And if they do happen to happen, you can fix them quickly.

I was once lucky enough to play golf at St Andrews in Scotland. And naturally, when I play golf I carry a fair bit of food with me, including fast-acting sugary sweets and drinks just in case I feel my levels dropping. But for whatever reason, on this particular day of all days, I was having real issues with my sugar levels. By about the 13th hole I had run clean out of all sources of sugar – including my playing partner's - and could feel the grip of hypo symptoms creeping up on me. I had to get my hands on some sugar quickly. I ended up wandering around the golf course like a zombie begging any passing golfer for the contents of their golf bag. I was lucky enough on the day to stumble across some very understanding Americans who passed over the sugary drinks they had happened to top up on before they started their round. They understood the situation and really helped me out. But I was lucky they were there. The clubhouse was over a mile walk away.

The moral of the story is of course to have a backup of sugar with you that will see you through any unforeseen situation. On that day I had no doubt under-eaten prior to starting out and had had way too much insulin with my pre-exercise meal. You will, like I did then and still do from time to time, get things wrong. You will under-eat or simply inject too much insulin. Carrying enough sugar to see you through these situations will help you prevent hypos from becoming more serious than they need to be.

Hypo Overeating

Hypo overeating is easy to do and definitely something I am guilty of from time to time. When you have a hypo, your instinct is to eat. And eat and eat. And to keep on eating until you feel better again. It's difficult to resist these urges when your sugar level is so low. But try to remember that it will take 15 minutes for the sugar you are eating to get in to your bloodstream. So if you keep on eating until you feel well again, remember that the food you have eaten over the last 15 minutes has still yet to get in to your system. By the time it does so, you will have fixed your hypo but you will have subsequently sent your sugar levels from being too low to being way too high.

This cycle is easy to get caught up in. We have a hypo, we overeat, we have a high sugar level, we increase our insulin injection and suddenly we have begun the cycle again. What you need to do is figure out exactly how much sugar you need to fix a hypo and get your sugar level back within the target band. For me, I know this is about half a bottle of a sugary drink. For you it may be something different. Trial and error is again the key. Try three glucose tablets and wait for 15 minutes. Then test your blood. Depending on how low your levels went, you will probably find you have got your levels back to over the 100mg/dL mark. If not then have a little more. You will quickly suss out how much sugar you need to get out of a hypo and back to where you should be. And when those hypo symptoms strike next time, try to stick to that same amount.

Chapter 7 – Alcohol

It's OK To Drink………Sensibly

Whilst I don't promote the idea of daily drinking episodes or of weekend binge drinking, most people drink alcohol and most will have the odd late night or two at the weekend. Nights out are an important part of our lives; especially when we are young. Some of our greatest friendships are forged from nights on the town and some of our best memories will be too. Being Type 1 Diabetic shouldn't take this away from you. As a Diabetic, it's important for you to drink safely and to be aware of the impact of alcohol on your sugar levels. Whatever age you are diagnosed at, drinking alcohol will most probably play a part in your life and you will have to learn how to fit your Diabetes around it.

You may well be reading this book before having reached the legal age to drink alcohol. If so then it is important for you to be armed with some decent knowledge about alcohol and Diabetes before you start experimenting with it. When I was diagnosed at the age of 14, I was given piles of pamphlets and magazines about my new condition. Everything I read seemed to want to scare me off from doing anything I wanted to do. Doctors would spend their time telling me what not to do rather than how to fit what I wanted to do around my Diabetes. Alcohol, smoking, drugs and anything else they deemed undesirable were simply regarded as things not to do. As if I would happily write them off and sit at home nursing my sugar levels for the next seventy years. That wasn't going to happen. Like most young people, I didn't like being told what to do. So I spent my teenage years doing what my friends and most other teenagers were doing.

Be Prepared

So, yes, you can drink. But you do need to be sensible about it. You are Diabetic and there are no days off. So, like it or not, everything you do will take a little planning and preparation. All the usual rules apply. Make sure you have a backup of sugar with you wherever you go. Take your pen and blood tester with you. And make sure that the people you are with know about your condition and what to do if you have a hypo. There is nothing you can't do, but you do need to plan everything you do much more than a non-Diabetic does. This is the reality – so get used to it.

In my late teens and early twenties I would be going out until morning to different clubs seeing various DJs do their thing. I was very much in to electronic music and everything that went along with the scene. Nights out could end up as weekends out – often ending up on a Sunday at some unplanned destination. I got away with it by having a good circle of friends around me who knew about my Diabetes and by carrying all my essentials with me wherever I went. Wherever I ended up, I would have my regular blood tests and I would have my insulin pen on me for meal times whenever they came around.

By no stretch of the imagination were my sugar levels constantly 100-160mg/dL throughout these weekends, but I did the best I could. And so will you. Teenagers and young adults have the worst average HbA1c test results of all the age groups. It's not ideal but it is a reality. Our sugar level management improves as we get older. As I have got older and my life has become a little more predictable, my sugar levels have in turn improved. The stats surrounding poor Diabetes management in younger people are indicative of the lifestyles they have. During your teens and early-twenties your life will not be consistent. Your college/university schedule may be different every day. You may not have a permanent job to go to Monday to Friday. You will be at parties, on nights out and your meal times will be more scattered than they should be. None of these things make for great management of your sugar levels but they are realities of your life and of growing up.

Nobody is giving you an excuse for being slack on your sugar levels. It's just a fact that a more moderate lifestyle makes it easier to control your Diabetes. But while you're young and out socialising, you can still look after yourself. Get used to taking your blood tester and pen to parties, to the pub or wherever you drink. Even when you are out drinking – especially when you are out drinking – you should be testing your sugar levels. You will learn soon enough the routine you need to follow to manage it as best you can. If you are going to be out around the time of your basal injection, set an alarm to remind you. And get your friends to nag you as much as they can to keep a check on your levels.

Avoid Buffering

Having to worry about your sugar levels on a night out can be trying. Always in the back of my mind when I am out drinking is whether or not my sugar level is slipping too low. Any time I want to go out and enjoy myself, I seem to get the little man on my shoulder checking up on me. I think I have always suffered slightly from an anxiety of having hypos – especially when out drinking or if I am out of my usual routine. So I always make sure my blood tester is close at hand. If I need to know, I can check. Having my blood tester with me reassures me everywhere I go.

An easy way of avoiding this Hypo Anxiety would be to buffer your sugar levels up so high that you don't have to worry about hypos for the night. I have to admit, I did this when I was younger. Instead of having to worry about my sugar level while I was out having a good time, I would reduce my mealtime injection a little. That way, my sugar level would be up around 200mg/dL for the night – or higher – and I wouldn't have to worry about having a hypo.

Needless to say, this buffering is a bad idea. The key to staying healthy with Type 1 Diabetes is to keep your sugar levels consistently within range. This shouldn't change just because you are out drinking alcohol. High sugar levels are bad and not something you should be doing to your body on a regular basis. Like it or not, you have to deal with looking after your sugar level, even when letting your hair down.

Try not to be scared of hypos. As a Type 1 Diabetic, they are inevitable. OK, they can be a bit of a nasty experience, especially when you are out trying to have a good time. But the odd hypo here or there, as long as you have your stash of sugar to hand, is preferable to going through life with constantly high sugar levels. Whilst drinking alcohol, you should treat your sugar levels the same as you do at any other time. Learn through trial and error. Figure out what is OK for you to drink and what isn't. Keep your blood tester with you so you can see which drinks affect your levels more than others. And, as usual, keep your friends close at hand so they can spot it if your sugar levels do begin to slip.

How Will Alcohol Affect My Levels?

Most alcoholic drinks contain sugar. When I go out these days – which is less often than when I was younger - I drink beer. I know that different beers have different quantities of sugar. I know because they affect my levels in different ways. Through quick blood tests after a few of a particular beer, I know which ones are the sugary ones and which ones aren't. And I order accordingly. Like the food I eat, I know how beer impacts my levels and I manage my levels as best I can. I would be more likely to achieve perfect sugar levels by staying home and not drinking, but I like going to the pub – so I go to the pub and fit in my Diabetes the best I can.

If I am drinking a certain amount of a certain drink, I will have a little bolus injection alongside it to stop my levels from going too high while I am out. This is not textbook stuff and is perhaps not advice that your doctor would give you. But the doctor and textbook would probably tell you to avoid the pub completely. Through experience, I know the impact certain drinks have on my levels and I know how many units of insulin will keep me within a decent range. Like everything, this has been a process of trial and error.

Beer is full with carbohydrates. So it's not actually a great choice of drink for a Type 1 Diabetic – especially in large quantities. What I do with beer is treat it like any other carbohydrate food. The food we eat is all measurable – we can count the carbohydrates we are consuming. Beer is no different. Through a bit of research we can find the rough carbohydrate values of a pint of beer. And we can measure the impact on our levels. An hourly blood test while out drinking will give you an idea of the impact it is having.

Different types of alcohol will have different impacts on your sugar level. I don't drink much wine but I have read that it doesn't have much of an effect on people's sugar levels. It certainly isn't as carbohydrate filled as beer. Spirits such as vodka or rum will be different again. The mixer may have more of an effect than the alcohol. Ultimately, you will only find out the impact of each drink once you have done some experimenting of your own.

From an early age, I was always told that alcohol lowers your sugar level. This certainly isn't true at the time of drinking it. The same as with food, if you drink something with sugar in it, your sugar levels will increase. But in the hours after drinking, your sugar levels can certainly drop. The carbohydrates in alcohol are generally of high GI value. This of course means that your blood sugar may crash a few hours after consuming it. So be careful, especially if you have been mixing alcohol with injections. It's important that, through testing, you get a good picture of what happens to your sugar levels during and after drinking alcohol.

Always test your sugar level when you get home. Although you may have tried your best, it's unlikely you will have a perfect sugar level after drinking alcohol. So take the chance to fix it before you get to bed. But be more careful than ever. Consider what you drank and, if anything, what you have already injected. You will need to, through blood testing, learn how your sugar level behaves in the hours after drinking.

Night time hypos can be dangerous – even more so after you have been drinking. If your sugar level goes low overnight and you don't wake up then you could have a big problem. This is the main reason that people may want to put Type 1 Diabetics off drinking at all. And it is the main reason why you have to be careful with everything you do concerning alcohol. While your liver is busy dealing with the alcohol you have consumed, it may not be able to release the necessary glucose you need if and when your sugar level begins to drop. This is the reality of the danger of hypos after drinking alcohol. If you do choose to inject to manage the carbs you are consuming in your alcohol then be cautious. Take time to understand the lasting effect of alcohol on your sugar levels and how a post-alcohol pre-bed time sugar level equates to a morning sugar level.

There is some rather obvious advice to give to you too. You should avoid sugary drinks. Don't drink Vodka and Coke – drink Vodka and Diet Coke. Cocktails will often have mountains of sugar in them. There are lots of mixers and bottled drinks that are stacked with sugar. Avoid these. Any drink with a high sugar content is of course not a good idea for you. Learn which drinks have the least impact on your sugar level and, if possible, stick to these.

Be watchful of your sugar level the day after drinking as well. I have often found that my levels will be lower the next day as my body works a little harder than usual in its efforts to recover. Put simply, I need to inject slightly less insulin on these days – maybe a unit or two fewer with breakfast and lunch. Whatever the science is behind this, it is something I have picked up on over time. There will be various quirks that you will discover to your own sugar levels. This is one I have discovered with mine. Everything you do and everything you eat will have an immediate impact on your sugar level and will probably have a lasting one too. Figure out what these are and adapt your regime to allow for them.

Choosing Not To Drink

There are of course lots of people all over the world who don't drink alcohol. Being alcohol-free is a healthier lifestyle choice whether or not you are Type 1 Diabetic. And if you do happen to be Diabetic, it is certainly a better way of looking after your sugar levels. As I get older, I certainly see the benefits to my weight, my sugar levels and to my general health and energy levels of drinking less alcohol and having fewer nights out. At the grand old age of thirty-five, rarely now will I be out past midnight. Life is easier as you get older, in many ways. A steadier, more conservative lifestyle is inevitable and your sugar level certainly sees the benefits.

So, if you choose not to drink then you will be doing your sugar levels a huge favour. But I wouldn't suggest to Type 1 Diabetics that they have to avoid it. You should go out and experience what you want to experience. Alcohol is often a part of being young and of bonding with your friends. You don't have to miss out just because you are Diabetic.

I am not telling all young people to go out getting drunk every night. But this chapter is an important one because, in reality, most people do drink and most young people diagnosed with Type 1 Diabetes will go on to experiment with various things in life – just like their non-Diabetic friends will. This will include alcohol. Nobody can or should want to stop you from doing that – but as a Diabetic you do need to take a lot more in to consideration that a non-Diabetic has to. Everything you do should be done so alongside a load of blood tests to figure out its impact on your levels. Once you've sussed that out then you should have a decent idea of how to go about doing it again whilst maintaining a decent grip on your Diabetes. Drinking, late nights and whatever else you get up to is included in that.

Whilst we accept them as part of life, nights out are a break from our usual routine. That's why we like them so much. But make sure they remain just that. If you are having three or four nights out drinking a week then it's unlikely that you will have a decent handle on your sugar levels. Your body may be able to handle a dodgy sugar level for a night. But it won't deal well with long-term bad management. So have fun but be healthy and sensible in all the decisions you make.

Chapter 8 – Checking Your Health

Finding Your Support Network

As a Diabetic it's great to have a team of people at your side to support you. Your support will come in many guises and of course should always begin with your friends and family. They should be the ones throwing chocolate at you when they see you sweating and the ones who nag you in to your pre-meal blood test. But there are experts at hand as well. Diabetic nurses, doctors and dieticians should all be a part of the support network you surround yourself with. You should use everything you have available to you. Although it is you who has to manage your Diabetes on a day-to-day basis, these extra sources of help should all come greatly appreciated.

With things in our lives that have become daily routines, we often struggle to see the woods for the trees. Our lives are routine – whether we like to think so or not. And the same is true with our management of Diabetes. We will get in to habits of eating the same breakfast, of buying the same foods at the supermarket and of eating the same stuff in the same restaurants. With this so often being the case, having the opportunity to report our routine to a diabetic nurse or to a dietician can be really worthwhile. These professionals see dozens of Diabetics like me and you come through their doors every week. That's a lot more than we may ever meet in our lives. They are able to pass on anecdotes and tips given to them by other Diabetics – on food, different types of insulins as well as new technology updates we might have otherwise missed. And some of this can be valuable information for us.

As a newly diagnosed Diabetic teenager, I was cynical of the advice given to me by these professionals. What did they know? They didn't have to inject themselves, have blood tests or to weigh their food out before they ate it. Who is this guy telling me what to do? I was angry that my life had been taken over by this condition and that doctors got to tell me what to do on the back of reading a textbook about it. However, as I got older and less angry about life, I started to listen a little more and realised there was some sound advice to pick up.

They may not be Type 1 Diabetic themselves, but they do know their stuff and are surrounded by the condition on a daily basis. Subjects I have covered already on Insulin, Carb Counting and the Glycaemic Index haven't come from books I have read. It has all come from face-to-face conversations with people I go to see every few months. I tell them what I am eating and when, how many units I am injecting and what I am doing day to day. In turn, they often pass on great nuggets of advice.

Try to set up a support network of your own. There are plenty of people out there who can help you so go for meetings as often as you can. Ask about what's going on in the world of Diabetes. What do they know that could help you out? I often leave with new food ideas or other tips of how to keep my levels steady. At worst, I will come away with a useful reminder to keep looking after myself.

HbA1c Tests

You will be tracking your daily sugar levels through your four or five finger prick blood tests. Finger prick blood tests are a great tool for you to use on a daily basis to track the impact of different foods and different insulin doses on your sugar level. But you also need to get an accurate idea of how you are doing over a longer period of time. That's why regular health checks are an important part of being Diabetic. Checking your levels over a longer period is the ultimate progress test of how you are shaping up as a Type 1 Diabetic.

Hba1c tests are something you should go and get regularly. Most doctors will recommend getting them done every three months. If you are newly diagnosed, maybe every couple of months. Once you are longer in the tooth and have your sugar levels more under control then doctors may lay off a little and suggest an Hba1c test every six months. Ultimately, it's down to you how often you have them. The more regularly you get it done, the more aware of your control you will be.

An HbA1c test will tell you how good (or bad) your sugar levels have been over the last eight weeks or so. And it's all to do with things called haemoglobin. Haemoglobin travels around your bloodstream carrying oxygen. The sugar in our blood, or glucose as we can call it, attaches itself to the haemoglobin as it circulates our body. The more glucose we have in our blood, the more of it that will attach itself to the haemoglobin.

When we have an HbA1c test, the nurse will stick a needle in our vein and extract some blood in to a tube. They will then take this blood off to a lab and count the amount of glucose attached to the haemoglobin. The amount of glucose that is found attached to the haemoglobin indicates the level of glucose in our blood over the last few weeks. Haemoglobin themselves generally survive in the bloodstream for around eight weeks. Therefore, counting the amount of glucose on each one gives us a pretty accurate idea of how much sugar has been in our blood over that duration of time.

So what is a good HbA1c level? Well, like with most things there are a couple of different ways of presenting the data. Results are sometimes recorded in mmol/l but are usually given as a percentage figure. The two are easy to convert from one to another. As a Type 1 Diabetic, you should be aiming for 7% or less as a score in your HbA1c test. Some people may tell you 6.5%. Of course it is relative. 8% is better than 9% and 6% is better than 7%.

A non-Diabetic will have HbA1c test scores of around 5%. So that is the ultimate, if somewhat idealistic, goal for a Type 1 Diabetic. Everyone will have their own expectations. But 7% and under is a good result for me. Hopefully over time I will continue to improve my sugar level management and will be able to reset my expectations.

As a newly diagnosed Type 1 Diabetic, your first few HbA1c test results will be nowhere near the recommended level. Don't worry too much – that's normal. But do make sure you do something about it quickly. A string of high HbA1c test scores will be doing your body some damage. I think my first couple were around the 10% mark. It was a sign of how difficult I found everything at the very beginning. Your first few months will be spent battling with your Diabetes as you just begin to gain some control over your levels. So don't be too hard on yourself in these first few months. But do make sure that every HbA1c result you get is better than the last one. You should aim to improve your levels gradually over time. Set yourself a target for when you will get it under 8%, under 7.5% and finally below the magic 7%.

When you are sent for your HbA1c, you will usually be asked to fast. That is to show up in the morning at the hospital without having eaten your breakfast. You can drink water before your blood is taken - but nothing else. The amount of time you should have actually fasted for is eight hours or more. This fasting is not specifically for your HbA1c test. When you go to get your blood taken, you may notice that they take two or three tubes from your arm, not just one. This is because they will be testing for some other stuff too.

They might, for example, test your cholesterol levels. To measure this, you will have had to have fasted. So make sure you check with the doctor what you are getting tested for and whether or not you will need to fast in advance of your blood test. And check again with the nurse who is taking your blood. They will probably ask you anyway – but make sure they know whether or not you have fasted for the blood test so they can give you accurate results of everything they test you for.

Why Do I Need to Have HbA1c Tests?

You need to have regular HbA1c tests to measure the overall control of your sugar levels. If you are checking in with regularly high HbA1c test results then it's an obvious sign that you haven't yet got your Diabetes under control. And you need to sort it out. Long term high sugar levels are bad news. HbA1c test results have been shown consistently to be a real barometer of a Diabetic's health. Improvement of your HbA1c results significantly decreases your chances of complications in the future. Results show that seemingly small improvements in your HbA1c test result do actually have a big impact on the likelihood of future complications. Reducing your score from 7.5% to 7.0% can make a significant impact on your future health.

So what of these 'complications' that people tell you about? Simply put, too much glucose in your blood will thicken it. Excessive glucose levels can also cause hardening of the blood vessels. These things cause circulation issues that can affect various parts of your body. Your feet and your eyes are two easy examples of things that can go wrong if you have consistently bad HbA1c scores. This is why when I visit the diabetic nurse, the first thing she does is whip my socks off and start prodding around at my feet. Sensitivity in your feet and toes are a sign that your circulation is still good. This is why your nurse will be sticking little pins in your toes – it's not because she doesn't like you.

Your internal organs can also be badly affected by long-term poor glucose management. *Hyperglycaemia* is the term used to describe high glucose levels. It can affect the functioning of your kidney, amongst other things.

This is why your doctor may also get your kidney functions checked whenever you go for your HbA1c test.

This isn't supposed to be a book designed to scare you in to looking after your sugar levels. Having already been diagnosed with Type 1 Diabetes, you have probably been warned about the dangers of hyperglycaemia and its long-term effects. Although it doesn't make for great reading, it is relevant and it is stuff you need to know about. The long and short of it is that looking after yourself and your sugar levels will allow you to live a long and relatively normal life. So keep healthy and try to be competitive with yourself with your HbA1c test results.

Retinopathy

You need to look after your eyes. In particular you need to look after your retina. The retina has tiny blood vessels that lead in to it. The blood flow through these is necessary for the whole thing to work and for us to see properly. So we will, every six months or so, be requested to go for a Retinopathy test. This test will zoom in on those blood vessels going in to the back of the retina. Thickened blood and hardened blood vessels can cause them to bulge – and in serious cases even to pop – affecting our eyesight. The Retinopathy test will look at those blood vessels and check to see if any are bulging or popping.

I go to get my retinas looked at every six months. I show up and before long I am called in to a room where someone puts drops in my eyes. I go back out, sit down and wait for twenty minutes or so. The purpose of these drops is to dilate the pupil so that those who know what to look at can get a good view of my retina. So after twenty minutes or so, everything is brighter than it was before and I am called back in to the room. I stick my chin on a strap and stare in to a machine. It takes photographs of my eyes. And that's it. I am sent home and I wait for a letter in the post with my results.

The drops that are put in your eyes dilate the pupil and will therefore mess with your vision a little – in particular your near vision. Reading a newspaper or a text message will be impossible for a couple of hours or so after the drops. For that reason, the doctors will always suggest that it's a bad idea to drive home from your appointment. So reach out to family and friends for a lift or go for public transport.

After twenty-one years of being Type 1 Diabetic, for me it is so far so good. I am by no means the perfect Diabetic. My retinopathy results sometimes tell me of small bulges in the blood vessels, but never of any signs of popping. But I must admit, the whole retina thing scares me and frequent tests are often the kick up the backside I need to keep my levels in check. That is really half the reason why I go to see the professionals as often as I can. I need reminders as often as possible to look after myself. Without seeing these doctors and nurses and getting the odd telling off then my levels can slip. A regular reminder to look after myself and my sugar levels is invaluable for me. After a grilling at the diabetic nurse or a letter from the retinopathy people, my levels are always good for a month or so. So these professionals are useful people. Go to see them as often as you can.

Be Your Own Doctor

It is great to get as many people around you as possible to help you with your Diabetes management. Seeing doctors, nurses and dieticians can never do you any harm. But ultimately you will be your own doctor. After a few months of living with your new condition, you will know more about your own Diabetes and your sugar levels than any professional can tell you. You will be the one monitoring your levels, figuring out your diet and your insulin doses. You will be the one who gets to know what sends your sugar level high and what might cause a hypo. You will know more about your own condition than anyone else and it is you who ultimately needs to take responsibility.

Having an ability to take a step back and reassess your diet, your insulin doses and your lifestyle is always great. Try to give yourself reviews. You don't always have to wait for the doctor or the dietician to tell you off. You can do that yourself. You don't always have to wait for a bad HbA1c test result to sort your sugar levels out. You should always have a good idea of how you are getting on and whether or not you have been doing the right things. So give yourself a monthly review. How have your levels been? What have you been eating? Where have your sugar levels been high? Do you need to change your insulin doses or the things you eat? Are you doing that thing the diabetic nurse told you to start doing last month?

For me, my motivation to keep on top of my Diabetes management lies in my own competitive instinct. I like to set myself targets. At the moment, I am trying to get consecutive HbA1c test results under 7.0. Other

Diabetics will have different goals. Whatever they are, set yourself some. Type 1 Diabetes is a numbers game. So figure out what you want yours to be and try to achieve your targets.

Chapter 9 – Progress in Technology

Insulin Pumps

I've already mentioned Insulin Pumps in this book. They are at the forefront of the technological progress that exists for Type 1 Diabetes. I remember when I first began to hear about them. Like everyone else, I was excited. It sounded like a replica pancreas. A fix. This is what I had been waiting for. But, for me at least, the excitement was short-lived. As soon as I began to find out more about them, honestly, I was disappointed. They weren't what I had hoped they were going to be. They weren't a replacement for my broken pancreas. Far from it. All they really do is help us to administer our insulin. Having said that, Insulin Pumps have been a hugely important invention for a lot of people around the world. Thousands of Type 1 Diabetics now have insulin pumps attached and it is an undeniable fact that this technology has reduced HbA1c test results for the vast majority of its users.

So what is an insulin pump and how does it work? Well, they are fundamentally an alternative to having injections. A small machine is stuck somewhere around your waist with a tiny needle attached to a catheter and placed under your skin. It releases bolus and basal insulin. The user digitally sets the basal dose for it to steadily release throughout the day. When it comes to meal time, you tell it how much bolus you want and it releases it for you. This is much like a normal bolus injection. You test your sugar level with a finger prick, count up your carbs and figure out how many units you need. The only difference here is that the pump is already attached to you. You don't need to have an injection.

So some people may prefer having a pump because it saves having injections. But it is by no means a replica pancreas. It doesn't decide how much insulin you have – you do. It doesn't stop your sugar level from going too high. It doesn't stop your sugar level from dropping too low. If you are lying on the ground having a hypo, it will still be releasing insulin in to you just like you told it to. Neither does it ever know what your sugar level is. You will only know this through your usual blood tests. Fundamentally, pumps are an alternative to you carrying your insulin around in a pen and injecting it.

So why all the fuss about insulin pumps? Well, the fact is that Type 1 Diabetics who convert from insulin pens to a pump do usually improve their Diabetes management and, therefore, their HbA1c scores. Statistics back this up. [1] A recent study in England showed that children switching from pens to pump improved their HbA1c scores by an average of 0.5%. But I don't necessarily want to give pumps the credit for this. Yes, they have proven to be a great asset for Diabetics who use them. And a pump might also prove to be a great decision for you too. But it isn't the pump that does the work. It is you. You decide your insulin doses

---

[1] https://t1dexchange.org/pages/insulin-pump-use-by-children-is-highest-in-us-collaboration-found/

and, of course, the food that you eat. Not your pump. But what your pump will do for you is give you a great reason to get on top of things.

The way I look at an insulin pump is as a symbol of your own commitment to you taking better care of your condition. Type 1 Diabetics who make the decision to attach an insulin pump to themselves are those who have already made that call. They have made the commitment – usually a financial commitment – to take good care of their sugar levels. They have invested in it. The pump will be there with you all day as a reminder to look after yourself; to manage your sugar levels properly and to think wisely about what you eat and about the insulin you are giving yourself.

This is how I explain the improvement in HbA1c test scores of those who choose to convert to a pump. The pump is not a magic wand. All it is doing is what you tell it to do. And your management of your sugar levels will only be as good as the decisions you make and the investment you make in it. Pumps have proven to be a great tool for a lot of Type 1 Diabetics. But, for me, they won't do anything your pens can't already do. It is you and your decision to manage your Diabetes closely that ultimately makes all the difference to your sugar levels.

This is why I have been a little disappointed in Insulin Pumps. They do nothing for me that my usual injections don't do - other than sit attached to me all day. Ideally, I want something that regulates my sugar level for me. This is what a functioning pancreas does. A working pancreas looks at the food you have eaten and releases the perfect amount of insulin to match it – keeping your sugar level consistently steady. And this is what I ultimately want from technology. So, the real question is, are we anywhere near getting technology to do this job for us? Can we have a machine that is continuously testing our sugar level whilst administering the right amount of insulin to keep our sugar levels in check? Are we anywhere near technology replicating the job of a pancreas?

CGM – Continuous Glucose Monitoring

Continuous Glucose Monitoring is amazing. Much like an Insulin Pump, it involves a little machine being strapped to your waist with a little needle stuck in to you. On this needle is a sensor. What it does is simple but truly ground-breaking, I think, for a Type 1 Diabetic. It tests your sugar level every five minutes and records it for you. It will send all of the data it gathers to your phone and make it available to you on an app. Now bear in mind that, without CGM, a good Diabetic will be testing their sugar level 5 times a day. A CGM machine tests your sugar level – wait for it – 288 times a day. Wow.

What CGM gives us is a 100% ability to understand our sugar levels. We can tell which foods were good and not good and which insulin doses were good and not good. It means we can track the impact of changes we make to our diet and our doses. It can tell us all about what our sugar levels do when we exercise. And it is there on our phone for us to glance at whenever we feel the need to know our sugar level. We can even get it to give us alerts whenever our sugar level has slipped too high or too low; allowing us to go about our daily lives whilst something else worries about what our sugar level is doing. Yes of course we still have to inject our insulin but, for me, that has never been an issue. If I am kept totally informed of what my sugar level does all day long, the insulin bit is made a lot easier.

Without CGM, a Diabetic might check their sugar level five times a day. So, we get a record of five moments in time during that day and what our sugar level was at each of those exact times. What we don't know is what our sugar level was at any stage between our tests. If I test my sugar level before lunch, it might be 150mg/dL. I then eat lunch and go about my day. Then, five hours later, I test my sugar level again before dinner and see that it is again at 150mg/dL. I now have information about where my sugar level was at two separate times of the day – five hours apart from one another. But what my levels were doing during that five hour period remains a mystery. It might have been 150mg/dL for the duration of that five hours. Or it could have risen to 250mg/dL after lunch, before dropping back down to 150mg/dL again before dinner. We don't know. CGM now removes this mystery.

CGM gives us a chart of our sugar level for every day we have it attached. We can see exactly the impact of each meal and how our sugar levels reacted at each part of the day. We can really see how different carbohydrates release in to our system. We can have detailed information about the impact of exercise on our sugar level. And all you need to do is attach it to yourself. This technology really is doing the hard part for us. The information CGM can give us on our sugar level is real gold dust for any Diabetic – Type 1 or Type 2.

But not so fast. There had to be a 'but' didn't there? The downside to CGM, as with many new technologies, is the cost. The cost of Diabetes and the availability of technology in general depends totally on where you live. In America, most people rely on their medical insurance to cover the costs of their Diabetes. And America is where most of the new technology is being used. In the UK, where I am from, I can get my insulin and test strips on prescription through the NHS, with the costs covered through our tax payments. But Insulin Pumps and CGM are not yet available through the NHS. In other countries across the world, the situation is totally different. Sadly, in a lot of poorer countries, there is no National Healthcare System and no Medical Insurance. There are a lot of Type 1 Diabetics in these countries who can't afford their insulin, let alone CGM or Insulin Pumps.

I have been in contact with some of the private companies who make the CGM technology available to buy. However, the cost is currently too high for me to get involved. CGM involves a sensor being attached to you for 24 hours a day. This sensor has to be changed – or it is recommended that it is changed – every 7 days. And it is the cost of these sensors that makes CGM technology out of reach for me, as well as for many others. The sensors are an expensive consumable. So, for me in the UK, without CGM being available on the NHS, the technology is a No Go. For the moment. I know it is only a matter of time before this and other successful technology becomes more mass produced and widely available. My hope is that it will soon be available to as many Diabetics as possible. Until then, I will keep badgering my NHS doctor about it. It is smart technology and could really make the ultimate difference in a lot of people's Diabetes management.

Future Technologies

So we have pumps that administer our insulin. And we have CGM machines that continuously measure our sugar level. I figure that, with these two things available, we are not far away from replicating the job of a pancreas. Surely all we need is for these two machines to talk to each other? We need the Insulin Pump to look at the readings of the CGM machine and administer the insulin we require to regulate our sugar levels. Much like a pancreas does. This combination would be the technology that I am looking for.

However, for the moment, this technology is not available. At least as I sit and write this, it is not available. I don't think we can be far off. What I recommend to you is that you keep yourself informed of what technology is out there. And what bits of it are available to you. Check the internet. Speak to your doctor, your diabetic nurse, your dietician and any other member of your support team. Compared to twenty-one years ago, there is so much out there. And there will be more within the next twenty-one years. As yet, we have no cure and no prevention for Type 1 Diabetes. But the technology becoming available to us can do a lot of the tough stuff for us. So get out there, see what is available to you, and take advantage of whatever you can get your hands on.

Apps and Stuff

We have covered Insulin Pumps and CGM. These are examples of life-changing technology for Type 1 Diabetics. And both are big decisions and big investments to make. They both involve having machines strapped to you 24 hours a day. But within technology, there is also smaller stuff that can make a big difference to your life.

On the app market you will find bundles of useful bits and pieces. I have apps that tell me about the Glycaemic Index value of the food I buy. There are also apps in to which I can scan barcodes to find out all sorts about the nutritional value of different foods. These kinds of things are great at educating us on the foods we need to be eating. And don't take it for granted just because it is available for free on an app. Be grateful. Just twenty-one years ago when I was diagnosed, nothing like this existed. There were a few books floating around doctor surgeries with sketchy information about carbohydrates and there were a few dieticians who might tell us what to eat and what not to eat. Nowadays we can really get a grip on what we are eating through the use of apps like this. It's easier to educate ourselves and, ultimately, to become our own doctor. I have a handful of apps I use on a daily basis to help me out with what I eat.

Also available on the app market are ways of tracking our sugar levels. CGM is able to do it for us – but isn't quite available to a lot of us yet. In its absence, we can stick to finger prick tests and use an app to track our levels. Using an app, we can quickly input our readings whenever we take them and it will begin to build a log of our entries. Of course, the more blood tests we have then the more useful the information that we get back will be. Apps can show us graphs of where our levels are before and after meals to help us identify any particular spikes or drops in our levels over time. This is really useful stuff. It can seriously help us with our Diabetes Management and help reduce our HbA1c scores. And it is available to us for free just by using our mobile phone.

Nothing Will Replace You

For all the talk of technology, it is still you who ultimately has responsibility over your sugar levels. The technology is great and is becoming more and more advanced. But if you aren't doing the right things as a Diabetic, no technology will be able to fix you. You need to eat the right food and you need to inject the right doses of insulin. No machine can make these decisions for you. But there are certainly lots of pieces of technology you can utilise along the way.

It is ultimately down to your decisions. Mainly it is about your decision whether to or whether to not take care of yourself. It is decision making that explains the improved HbA1c test results of Insulin Pump users. The psychological investment required to have a pump fitted is a sure sign that that Diabetic intends to take their condition seriously. And the HbA1c test results for pump users are undeniable. Once they have that pump fitted, they are invested in managing their condition. The same can and hopefully will be true of CGM. It will give you unreal levels of information about what affects your sugar level and how. But it will still be up to you to do something about it.

So educate yourself on the technology that is available to you and go and get whatever you think will help you. There is no one way to manage your condition. Only you will know what is best for you and for your lifestyle. Some people may want to be hooked up to a pump. Some may not. Different solutions will suit each person's lifestyle. And don't forget that, for all the technology you might want to use, it is still you who carries the can on your sugar levels. Not a machine.

Chapter 10 – Finding the Balance

The Battle

I feel like there is a constant battle going on as a Type 1 Diabetic. The battle between Looking after your Diabetes and Having a Life. Of course it is possible to have both. But it is a battle and we do have to strike some kind of balance. As a Diabetic you have to consider everything you do more than a non-Diabetic does. Everything you do. Meal times, going swimming, going out for lunch, going to the cinema, playing sport, going on holiday. All this stuff needs careful consideration as to how we are going to fit our meals and our injections around them.

How am I going to manage my sugar levels? How much insulin will I need if I am doing that afterwards? Will I need to take extra food with me? Do I have enough insulin to last me? How many test strips do I have in that box? Where are we going to eat breakfast? Will they have sugar-free drinks? These are all the questions I start asking myself whenever a plan is being made. It sounds obsessive. But we do have to be a little obsessive about our Diabetes to be able to manage it properly.

Being Organised

Managing our Diabetes every day can get stressful. But I find decent preparation is less stressful than being out and about somewhere and not knowing where my next meal is coming from or what my sugar level is. I organise everything I do to make sure I am able to fit in my Diabetes around it. I used to have a job that involved a lot of travel to other countries and to other continents. Whenever I went abroad I would insist on organising the whole thing. I think people just assumed I was a control freak. (That might not be completely inaccurate.) But really it was so I could plan my schedule and my meals properly. I didn't want to have breakfast at 7am and then wait until 3pm to eat my lunch. I just didn't want to have to be reaching for the emergency packs of sugar during meetings or during flights. If I knew when and where I was eating I would be relaxed and able to do my job. A Diabetic with an empty belly is never on top form.

So my tip is to be organised. Have a good idea of where and when you are going to eat each day. Space your meals out. If you are away from home for a while, make sure you take the essentials with you. Your insulin, your blood tester and your stash of sugar. With the Diabetic Trinity by your side you won't go too far wrong. Make sure others know you are Diabetic and that meal times are important. This can be more difficult. I feel uneasy dictating to other people. But I do need to eat at certain times so I will do it when it comes to food. I find that people will generally cut you some slack if you explain to them why meal times are important to you. For me, lack of organisation just leads to inconvenient hypos and all round bad days. You can avoid these with some basic preparation in everything you do.

Having a Life

Being organised doesn't mean you have to say No to everything. It just means you need to take ten minutes to prepare what you are doing before you set about doing it. You could say No to everything and sit at home all day nursing your sugar levels. But please don't do that. I try to make a point of doing everything I can; if only to prove to myself that I can do it. And to prove to my Diabetes that it's not going to stop me from enjoying myself.

Don't let your Diabetes keep you prisoner to any extent at all. Make it inspire you to do more. Make sure you exercise. Make sure you have fun, travel, do what you want to do. Fit your Diabetes around your life. Don't make your whole life about being Diabetic.

There are times when your sugar level will be too high. And you will have hypos. But Type 1 Diabetes is not about having perfect sugar levels all day. At least, I don't think it is. It is about being on top of it while you get on with living your life. Set your standards high in terms of managing your sugar level because being healthy will give you a quality of life. But also be realistic. You will rarely achieve perfection with Type 1 Diabetes.

If I play sport, my sugar levels will be imperfect. If I go out for dinner, my sugar levels will be imperfect. If I go travelling or do anything else that might stretch my comfort zone, my sugar levels will definitely be imperfect. That is part of living life as a Diabetic. Yes, better HbA1c test results do directly affect your health. So make sure each score you get is the absolute best you can make it. But don't let it be a reason for you to stop doing the things you want to do.

Travelling

For me, being Diabetic is a challenge. It can actually inspire me to do things that maybe I wouldn't ordinarily have done. Having freedom to do whatever I want is absolutely the most important thing to me. And my Diabetes certainly doesn't stop me from having it. Travel is important to me too. I love being on aeroplanes and adventuring in different countries. I was lucky that my previous job saw me travel to countries all around the world. Outside of work, I have travelled around Europe and around South East Asia.

Everywhere I have gone has needed some serious planning. And every day I have been away has needed some organisation to manage my levels properly. I have had to take away pretty large quantities of insulin with me to some of the places I have been. Getting through customs with three months worth of insulin, needles and test strips has sometimes required some explaining. But, up until now at least, nobody has tried to take it off me or stopped me from getting to where I am going. I have had to spend a day rummaging around chemists in Asia trying to buy basal insulin after unexpectedly running out. Things you do sometimes need a little bit of extra work when you're Diabetic. But for me it all adds to the challenge and to the adventure.

Eating abroad can be difficult too. I can plan to eat at the right times. I can have lunch on time. It's easy enough to manage my own schedule when I'm travelling. But the food is more out of my control. In many of the places I have been to abroad, I am eating food cooked at the side of the road. I eat it sitting on a plastic stool or on the pavement. There is no menu, no ingredients list. There is certainly no barcode to scan. So guessing the insulin dose is often just that – a guess. But this is life. I could sit at home and scan all my barcodes and achieve amazing HbA1c tests every three months. Or I can go out, travel and live my life; fitting in my Diabetes around what I want to do. Sometimes I will get my insulin dose wrong. Sometimes my sugar level will be too high. Sometimes I'll have a hypo. But this is life as a Diabetic. Your sugar levels won't be perfect all of the time. And if they are, maybe you are not doing all the things you could be doing.

So you have to do the best you can. And wherever you are, whatever you are doing, you can achieve good control. Make sure you have five blood tests a day. There is never anything stopping you from doing that. I ran clean out of test strips while I was travelling once. I couldn't get the same ones that fitted my meter in any chemist. So I bought a new blood tester and a supply of new test strips. I had to change some stuff around but I could still have my blood tests. Five blood tests a day will ensure that any highs or lows will be corrected quickly. You will have peaks and troughs when you are out of your routine, but regular testing can make sure they are short-lived.

Always take your insulin with you wherever you go. Like I have said, in the UK keeping it cool is not even a consideration. It's always cool - at best - in the UK. But when I have travelled I have had to take some steps to make sure I look after my insulin and stop it from heating up too much. There are plenty of insulated little bags you can buy for this kind of thing. So get hold of one if you are ever going anywhere hot.

Another thing I have come to learn about travelling abroad is that, along with the trinity of your insulin, blood tester and sugar stash, you should always carry a copy of your prescription. This can help in airports and also at chemists where you may need to buy some back up supplies. Remember that Type 1 Diabetes is not so common in a lot of countries. In South-East Asia, for example, they have plenty of cases of Type 2 Diabetes but a very small number of Type 1s. Most people are not aware of Type 1 at all. So when I, a relatively healthy looking 35-year old guy, tell people in these places that I am Diabetic, it often causes confusion. "But you're young." "But you're not fat." They assume I am Type 2 because this is all they know. But having a copy of my prescription handy, although it doesn't always completely solve the confusion, makes it clear what it is I need to get hold of.

There's Nothing You Can't Do

When planning to write this book, I wanted to make it different from some of the medical-based stuff that might have been given to you when you got diagnosed. A lot of what I was given when I was diagnosed gave me the impression that there was stuff that I wasn't allowed to do anymore. That's also how a lot of non-Diabetics seem to think about it. Like we have some kind of allergy. But Type 1 Diabetes isn't an allergy. I don't really see it as a disease either. It's a condition and it's a way of life. And it is your way of life. There is nothing you are not allowed to do.

Yes, you do have to fit your Diabetes in to every day you live. This becomes our routine. It's important to keep our sugar levels steady. It's important to eat the right foods, to take the right insulin doses. It's important to get regular checks at the doctors. You never get a day off as a Diabetic. But none of this really stops you from doing anything. And don't let anyone else tell you otherwise. Everything you do will take extra planning – that much is true. But there are great examples all over the world of Type 1 Diabetics doing amazing things; maybe things they might never have done if they didn't feel like they had a little extra to prove to themselves.

Ultimately, managing your Diabetes is all about finding your balance. It's about fitting your Diabetes around all the things you want to do in your life. Achieving everything you want to whilst maintaining good management of your sugar levels is totally possible. So don't sit at home nursing your pen and your blood tester. Take them out in to the wild and give them some tales to tell.

Chapter 11 – Perceptions and Misconceptions

The Diabetes Mystery

I always feel like there is a bit of mystery surrounding Diabetes. A lot more so than there should be or than there needs to be. Thousands of us live with this condition every day of our lives but, to be honest, not many of the people around us really understand what it is. And the average guy in the street I try to explain it to can't get his head around it either. But what's not to get? You have a pancreas. When you eat, your pancreas releases insulin to regulate the amount of sugar going in to your blood. Mine doesn't work. So I have to do that job manually through a careful mix of diet and insulin injections. That's how I explain it to people. I think that's a decent enough explanation. But I still get asked the same nonsensical questions in response.

"So is it the one where you have to eat sugar or have you got the one where you're not allowed to eat sugar?"

"Do you have to have injections every day or just some days?"

"What happens if you eat chocolate? Do you have a fit?"

"My mate has Diabetes and he has to eat 4 Mars Bars a day."

Let's be honest. As a Type 1 Diabetic you are going to hear a multitude of dumb questions. There is a genuine ignorance about it. It still amazes me the stuff that people come out with about, what I believe to be, a very simple condition. A part of our body doesn't work. So we have to do its job manually. Or maybe I'm just explaining it wrong.

Type 1 vs Type 2

OK so we know about Type 1 Diabetes. We know what it is, how it happens, how it works. So what is this Type 2 that everyone goes on about? Apparently there is a worldwide epidemic. We certainly hear enough about it on the news. Well, Type 2 Diabetes is different from Type 1 in the way it comes about. The most important thing to understand is that Type 2 Diabetes is not an auto-immune condition. It has nothing to do with the immune system attacking the pancreas. But Type 2 Diabetes is related to insulin levels and it does ultimately have the same effects, if badly managed, as Type 1.

In Type 1 Diabetes, the immune system attacks the pancreas and renders it unable to produce any more insulin. This is not the case with Type 2 Diabetes. In fact, most Type 2 Diabetics have a functioning pancreas that still produces insulin. But the levels of insulin created in a Type 2 are not high enough to be able to successfully regulate blood sugar levels. Type 2 can also be caused by insulin resistance which is when the body is unable to use the insulin it creates effectively enough to control sugar levels.

So is Type 2 Diabetes 'fixable'? Well, sometimes it can be successfully managed through an improved diet. Sufferers are often able to control their sugar levels by adopting a new, healthier, low carb diet. If the carbs they are putting in to their body are manageable with the low amount of insulin they produce then they will be able to keep their sugar levels under control.

Lots of people ask me why their Gran or their Uncle has been diagnosed as Type 2 Diabetic. If, as they have got older, their pancreas is not functioning at 100% anymore, it may be struggling to produce the required level of insulin. If this is the case then it may not be able to produce enough insulin to be able to regulate the blood sugar levels effectively. Again, this will cause hyperglycaemia and will be labelled as Type 2 Diabetes. So is this one fixable? Well, again it can be controlled by diet. If the sufferer can lower their carbohydrate intake enough to match the amount of insulin their pancreas is still creating, then they will be able to control their blood sugar levels. Again this is down to a new, healthier and much stricter diet. However, if the pancreas just isn't creating enough insulin to keep sugar levels under control then some small insulin injections may be necessary to successfully regulate the sugar levels. So, yes, some Type 2 Diabetics may also have to inject insulin.

It is a fact that there are way more Type 2 Diabetics around today than there were fifty years, or even twenty years ago. But how much of this is down to an 'epidemic' and how much is down purely to increased diagnosis of the condition? It is possible that a big proportion of this increase is increased diagnosis rather than actual increases in cases of Type 2 Diabetes. The word 'epidemic' is actually a horribly misleading and lazy expression used by media to talk about Diabetes. It suggests Type 2 Diabetes is something we are all catching from one another. This word and other ways in which Type 2 Diabetes is reported don't help the myths and ignorance surrounding the condition. Yes, we do have a lot more sugar in our diet than we did years ago. And yes this is bad. And yes it will put a strain on our pancreas and cause more cases of Type 2. But it does seem these days that everyone and his dog is a Type 2 Diabetic.

The Confusion

"Oh yeah, my Gran's got that."

There has been a huge surge in the number of Type 2 Diabetics in recent years. Something like 90% of all Diabetics are now Type 2 Diabetics. And this totally confuses most people. A lot of people will associate Diabetes with that thing their Gran was told she had a couple of years ago. And now their Gran isn't allowed to eat biscuits anymore and has to put sweeteners in her tea instead of sugar. But sometimes she still has sugar in her tea because she likes it or because she forgets and then she feels poorly. Is that what you've got then?

This is the common story I get from people when I tell them that I'm Diabetic. If I explain that I'm Type 1 not Type 2 then it doesn't seem to help.

"Oh right, so you've got the one where you need sugar. Right?"

Well, no it's not like that at all. When we try to explain to people about our Type 1 Diabetes, it confuses them. The condition we explain doesn't fit what they have heard about on the news or read about in the papers. News stories on the TV about cases of Type 2 Diabetes will be loosely referred to as being about 'Diabetes.' They will show fact sheets on screen about 'Diabetes' cases increasing and treatment for 'Diabetes' when what they are actually specifically referring to is Type 2 Diabetes. The reporting we have seen over the past decade or so certainly hasn't helped the cause of us minority Diabetics – the Type 1s.

The over-simplification in the media of Diabetes creates total misunderstandings about it in the general public. Much like any other subject in the media, we are fed over-generalised and often plain misinformed stories and statistics about Diabetes. The news or the newspapers will often be the first exposure the average person will get to the condition. People will watch it, listen to it, read about it and store the information given to them in their head as their titbit of knowledge on the subject. This is how the media works and this is how our heads work. The first actual Diabetic the average person will meet or hear about will also - 90% chance - be a Type 2 Diabetic. The information received in this encounter will reaffirm their previously gained knowledge on the subject of Diabetes. So it's little wonder then that when we meet them and start telling them all sorts of stuff about being a Type 1 Diabetic, we are so often met with puzzled faces.

The Postcode Lottery

Knowledge of Type 1 Diabetes varies dramatically depending on where you are. It is quite a geographically centralised condition. What I mean is, it is far more common in some areas than in others. Northern Europe and North America have the highest rates. The US, Canada, the UK, Scandinavia and Australia have the highest incidents of Type 1 Diabetes in children. In these areas, at least 2 in every 10,000 kids aged 0-14 are diagnosed with Type 1 Diabetes each year. This roughly equates to two kids in each school being Type 1 Diabetic. Across Asia and Central and Southern America it is comparatively rare (less than 0.4 cases annually per 10,000 kids)[2].

This makes being Type 1 Diabetic in some of the places mentioned incredibly difficult. In many countries around the world, health services don't have the facilities and support network that is afforded to us in UK, in Europe, Australia and North America. We are lucky in our rich western countries. Despite the confusion between different Types of Diabetes, the condition is largely known about here. It is also supported through various public or private health systems. In other – often poorer - parts of the world, the condition is rare, has no medical funding from governments, and is just not known about. This means that life expectancy for a kid diagnosed with Diabetes in these poorer countries is much shorter than in countries of higher incidents. They miss out on the knowledge of

---

[2] http://www.diapedia.org/type-1-diabetes-mellitus/21040851118/geography-of-type-1-diabetes

the condition and sometimes on the basic availability of manufactured insulin. Sadly, Type 1 Diabetes can be a terminal illness for a lot of kids in poorer countries. In time I would like to think we can do something about this and make sure every kid diagnosed with Type 1 Diabetes has the same support network and facilities available to them - irrespective of the country they are born in.

Travelling around Asia in particular really showed me how little anyone knows about Type 1 Diabetes. Type 2 is becoming more widespread in Asia. This is down to increased capabilities of diagnosis but also conceivably down to an increasingly sugary diet as Western brand names and foods begin to flood the East. But they don't call it Type 2 – they just call it Diabetes. That is the only sort they know. So when I try to explain to new friends in Asia about my condition, they assume I am Type 2 – like their Gran. They are baffled. They think it's my fault. They think that if I eat more healthily then it will go away. I get disapproving looks like I have done something bad.

"But you're not fat."
"But you're not old."
"He must eat too many sweets. Give him some fruit and he'll be alright."

I always find it odd that people's solution to me having Diabetes is to give me food. They are confused and I am frustrated in not being able to get my message across. Then we eat together and I start sticking needles in myself and then they go away. New friends lost.

So What Should We Call It?

You might have picked up on my sense of frustration – annoyance even – around the confusion that is Diabetes. In particular about the rising awareness of Type 2 confusing people as to what Type 1 actually is. I am happy to say that I am not alone. In an attempt to allay confusion, there is a call from Type 1 Diabetics to change the name of Type 1. As I write, there exists a petition with 15,000 names on it[3]. Many of the names on there are those of mothers who are fed up with the misconceptions people have of their Diabetic son or daughter. These misconceptions are real and are becoming more common.

Switching on the news and hearing about the rising cases of Diabetes being caused by poor diets and obesity annoys me. And it annoys a lot of Type 1 Diabetics. Our condition was not caused by having a poor diet or by being obese. And no amount of exercise or improved diet will ever be able to cure it. Neither could it ever have prevented it. The use of the word 'Diabetes' is loose at best by the media and, I am afraid, will cause people confusion about your condition wherever you go.

So what should we call Type 1 Diabetes? Do we really need to rename it? Well, there have been a few suggestions and there are a few already commonly used. Of those already used to define Type 1 Diabetes, *Juvenile Diabetes* has been perhaps the most common. Type 1 is

---

[3] https://www.change.org/p/revise-names-of-type-1-2-diabetes-to-reflect-the-nature-of-each-disease

often referred to as Juvenile Diabetes because of when most cases are diagnosed. The vast majority of Type 1 Diabetics get their condition somewhere between the ages of 1-15 years old[4]. I was relatively late when I was diagnosed at the age of 14. Again, we don't know why this is. We don't know why we get it as a kid. We don't know why the immune system does what it does and we don't know why it chooses childhood as the right time to do it. But it does give us a decent way of defining the condition. Juvenile Diabetes is an OK way of distinguishing Type 1 from Type 2. But it is not consistently used. Neither does it account for the rising number of Type 1 cases in adults.

The blurring of the lines between Type 1 and Type 2 has made the use of other terms more difficult. As has the increase in the number of adults being diagnosed with Type 1. But it is generally agreed that more education on and more awareness of the different types of Diabetes would be a good thing. A change in the terms we use to describe the different Types would no doubt aid that.

The term *Insulin Dependent Diabetes* is also now somewhat redundant. Many Type 2s require low levels of additional insulin to help them with their sugar level management. Others take tablets. Some sources will tell you that, if you inject insulin, then you are Type 1; regardless of whether your Diabetes was caused by an auto-immune condition or not. This confuses the situation even more. And as the lines of Type 1 and Type

---

[4] https://myglu.org/articles/a-focus-on-key-findings-age-of-diagnosis-and-a1c

2 continue to blur together, we are all a bit lost for proper definitions.

None of this is to suggest that Type 1 is necessarily more 'serious' than Type 2. That isn't my point or anyone else's point. The 'seriousness' of your Diabetes, whichever Type you happen to be, is dictated purely by your own management of it. A Type 1 Diabetic with good management of their sugar levels will always be healthier than a Type 2 Diabetic with poor management. But for clarification of your condition and what other people should know about it, I and many others hope that some more descriptive terminology can soon be used.

The long and short of this chapter is that people will be confused about your Diabetes. That's what you need to be aware of. People I speak to generally are. I have given up trying to articulate it and often just refer people to websites to go away and read. Some are interested and some aren't. Many are still confused. But it is important that those around you – your friends and family – are interested and that they understand your condition. They need to appreciate that it is something you will have every day for the rest of your life. They need to understand that there was nothing you did to cause it and that there is nothing you can do to make it go away. And they need to understand that your Diabetes is different to what their Gran has. Those who care will listen, watch, understand and you can add them to the support network you will go on to build around yourself.

Chapter 12 – Knowing Other Diabetics

Talk About It

My biggest regret of my twenty-year stretch as a Diabetic is that I have never really interacted with other Diabetics. As a newly diagnosed teenager, my doctor kept on telling me that he was organising a monthly get-together for kids like me to meet up and share our experiences. But it never materialised. The thing about kids – and teenagers in particular – is that they are shy. As a fourteen year-old kid, shy, moody and not over the moon about my new situation, the idea of a monthly meet-up sounded pretty unappetising. At the time, I just wanted someone to give me what I needed, tell me what to do, then go away and let me get on with it. The range of emotions most young people go through when they are diagnosed doesn't often lead to them sharing their struggles with it.

In hindsight, the opportunity to meet up with people of my age and in the same situation would have been invaluable. I struggled with my Diabetes for a long time and was pretty miserable about it. This was in the days before mobile phones and before the internet. There was nothing on TV about Diabetes and nowhere to get much information about it. The only real interaction I had with people was when I went to see the doctors and diabetic nurse every few months and get told off about my HbA1c test results. The only things I had to read were some sterile looking pamphlets handed out to me at the hospital telling me not to smoke or to do drugs. And I turned down the only hope of interaction with another human.

From what I know, there were two Diabetics in our school of around 1,200 kids. About the national average. When I got back to school after a week in the hospital, my teacher asked me whether I wanted her to organise a meeting with a guy in the year above me who had been Diabetic for a few years. I said No. I don't know why. I suppose I was shy and wasn't ready to talk to people about it. But I know this was a chance missed. It was also an opportunity for the other guy to share his own experience – which he might well have appreciated doing. Up until then he had been the only Diabetic kid in the school and would have been as devoid as me of opportunities to compare stories. Ultimately it was a chance missed for the both of us.

I didn't really sort my Diabetes out for a long time. I went through all of my school and subsequent university years managing my levels pretty poorly. I had never reached out to any other Diabetics nor bumped in to any. I was still on two injections a day – a mixture of bolus and basal – and found it difficult to fit it all around my life. Frankly, as most young people do, I had other priorities at the time. Looking after my Diabetes was not top of my list. But I was still having my HbA1c tests and going for regular tellings off at the doctors. This kept me in check to a certain extent.

It was only when I was 22 years-old, having been Type 1 Diabetic for eight years, that I started to look after it a lot more carefully. I had a job and a regular routine. My daily routine, more than anything, helped me get on top of my levels. Having breakfast, lunch and dinner around the same time every day made it much easier for me to control my levels. It was certainly a total contrast to my university days. The other thing I changed, and not before time, were my injections. I finally got on to having four injections a day. One basal and three bolus injections. My sugar levels saw an instant improvement.

Using The Internet

It can be lonely out there for a Type 1 Diabetic. Newly diagnosed and without anyone to bounce ideas off, you are left alone to battle with this new and somewhat befuddling condition. But help is always at hand. Communication and the sourcing of information has been revolutionised in the last 20 years by the internet. We suddenly have far fewer excuses for feeling alone. There is a tonne of information available to you online. The most valuable thing the internet gives you is instant access to a load of people in the same situation as you. It's not difficult these days to go online and share your ideas and your problems with other Diabetics all across the world. The internet really is an amazing tool and, as a Diabetic, you should be using it.

There are hundreds of websites that can be useful to a Diabetic – all easily locatable through your usual search engine. So take a look and find your own favourites. There is information on different types of insulin, on glycaemic contents of food and on Carb Counting. You name it, it's out there. There are Diabetic cooking guides. Anything you want or need to know about food can be found online. It's also great for keeping up-to-date with new technology. I use the internet regularly to check up on CGM and when I might be able to get my hands on it. Whatever technology you are interested in, and wherever you live, information is always at your fingertips.

There are some useful books out there to read too. Hopefully including this one. Books are the #1 sold item on the internet. So get on there and have a look for books you might find useful. eBooks can be downloaded at the click of a button. There are books on everything you might need to know about, from life with an insulin pump to guides on cooking and carbs.

Message boards are the most useful tool available to you as a Diabetic. This is your opportunity to share your experiences and to hear about how other people are managing their sugar levels. Type 1 Diabetes is not a common condition. I have only ever come across a handful of people with it; none of whom I regularly keep in contact with. But finding them on the internet is a piece of cake. Jump on to one of the many Diabetes message boards and you will find hundreds of Diabetics just like you to share information with. Some of them have been Diabetic for years and some are recently diagnosed. Some will be good at managing it and some not so good. Spend some time in these places and you will quickly pick up tips on what to do and what not to do.

Always remember to give as well as take. Any ways you have found to reduce your HbA1c scores will be useful to others. There are thousands of people all over the world who are just like you. You might not bump in to them on the street but you will find them online. This is a reassuring thing to realise and it is also an opportunity for you to help others. They too will be searching for better ways to do things; better foods to eat and insulin regimes to follow. So share your experiences with anyone you can. Start a blog. Do anything you can to increase the knowledge base for Diabetics and for those people who live with Diabetics. It's great to find people who have the same questions as you and who go through similar things each day. You may also find the internet to be a useful place to vent to people who might understand your problems a little better than your friends and family do.

Get Some Face-to-Face Contact

What I have really lacked in my time as a Diabetic is face-to-face encounters with other Diabetics. I get the impression that not many of us are blessed with this opportunity. I actually regret not holding on to some of the other Diabetics I have met. Even if they aren't going to be your best friend, even if you share no other interests, it's good to have that face to share your experiences with. I have always found that there is not much in place for us to do this. Or maybe I'm not looking hard enough. Either way, it doesn't stop you or I from setting something up. Your Diabetic Nurse will meet many more Diabetics each week than you maybe will in a lifetime. Use that contact to see if you can get to meet up with other Diabetics. If there is nothing already in place for face-to-face sharing, then try to set something up. A monthly gathering of Type 1 Diabetics would be useful for a lot of other people out there.

However you want to do it, you have all the means necessary to share your experience with others. And be grateful for what you have at your fingertips. It wasn't long ago that Diabetics had nothing but pig insulin to try to survive on. Before that there was not much at all. Even at the time of my diagnosis, there were very few ways of getting or sharing good information on what I was supposed to be doing with my condition. But technology has brought us a long way. We have Insulin Pumps, Continuous Glucose Monitoring, manufactured insulin and accurate blood sugar readings whenever we want them. And there is more and more technology coming around all the time. But the internet could be our greatest tool of all – so go and use it.

Chapter 13 – Be Your Own Diabetic

Every Type 1 Diabetic is different. We all have unique bodies, different diets and different lifestyles. It's great to read books, to get advice and to share experiences. These are your tools and sources of information necessary for you to improve your HbA1c scores. But ultimately your Diabetes will be yours to manage. Nobody will do the hard work for you. And what works for one Diabetic may not work for another. An appropriate insulin dose for one may be inappropriate for another – even if you are eating the same meal. So there is a load of amazing support out there for you. But there are no set rules.

Having spoken to a handful of other Diabetics, I realise that we are all on completely different insulin doses. These days those who inject are generally on four injections a day. One basal and three bolus. But we are all on different amounts. Someone of the same sex, age and weight as you might eat the same food as you and do all the same things; but you will still be on different doses of insulin. I don't have any science to explain this. I can only tell you that we are all different and the best regime for someone else will not necessarily be the best option for you. There are different manufacturers of insulin. There is an endless supply of different foods for you to eat. We all have different jobs and different hobbies. All of these variables lead to you having a unique condition.

You should share your experience with other Diabetics so we can learn from each other. You should use your support network of doctor, diabetic nurse, dietician and whoever else you have. You should get as many checks on your HbA1c, your feet, your eyes and whatever else as you possibly can. But, even after all this, the only person that is going to look after you is you. You are the one who decides what food to eat, what drinks to drink, what exercise to do as well as every other decision in your life that will affect your sugar level management. How you feel about this is up to you. You have total control and responsibility over your sugar levels. If they are healthy then it's because of your good management. If they are unhealthy then it's because of your bad management. That's how it is. You're in control.

Type 1 Diabetes is a condition you carry around with you everywhere you go. There are no days off. This is something we come to accept and get used to. But it is a total pain in the arse. That's the only way I have ever been able to describe it. It is of course possible for you to live a long and healthy life just like everyone else. You just have to work a bit harder at it. But maybe that makes it more rewarding. There are things in all of our lives that we have done - achievements that we have made – that were inspired by some kind of adversity. It is in our nature to stick two fingers up at hardship and to go out and prove it wrong. This is the best way to think about Type 1 Diabetes. Don't let it stop you from doing everything you want to do in your life. Make it the inspiration behind the things you achieve. Us other Diabetics need people to look up to.

Like anything in life, you will have good days and bad days. Good months and bad months. Some months I find my sugar levels easy to keep on top of. But sometimes it just doesn't want to behave. My sugar level seems to do inexplicable things sometimes. It will go through the roof for no apparent reason. All we can do in these situations is fix it. And regular blood testing will ensure that no high or low sugar level will stay that way for long. So you won't always have a perfect sugar level. If you are living any sort of a life then it's near impossible. The key is to make your management as good as possible. Fit it around your life the best you can. And keep improving it. Keep on sharing and learning. You should be able to improve it year after year as you begin to master it. I have been Type 1 Diabetic for twenty-one years and am nowhere near Master status – but my HbA1c tests are steadily falling as I get older and wiser.

Most of us get Diabetes as a youngster. What that means is that your condition will change and evolve over the coming years as your body continues to grow. In reality, our body never stops evolving. And all of these changes will affect our sugar levels too. As your body grows older, your metabolism will change. In general it will slow down. This will affect the rate at which the carbs you are eating enter your bloodstream. So you will have to adapt your regime to suit it. It is a constantly moving target. You will find that your trial and error of different foods, different insulins and different doses never ends. You will constantly need to make changes here and there to your management to keep on top of the changes going on in your body.

Be competitive with yourself. If you have Diabetic friends who you can share the competition with then great. My usual quarterly goal is to achieve a lower HbA1c than the last one. I might sound like a Diabetes geek but I'm not. I just know I need to have goals to achieve in life. Of course, I don't always achieve them. But I do find that, over a twelve month period, I generally lower my average from the previous year.

I hope the theme of this book has been apparent enough. Just in case you missed it, my message is to fit your Diabetes around doing all the things you want to do in your life. Not the other way around. Own it. Don't let it own you. As I type this, I am sitting in my little office in Hanoi, Vietnam, overlooking West Lake. What am I doing here? I often ask myself that question. Well, I like to seek out new challenges in life in an attempt to widen my once very small comfort zone. Two years ago, that led me to buying a one-way ticket to South-East Asia. I wanted to know if I would survive. It was my new challenge. I wanted to prove to myself I could do anything I wanted to do. So I quit my job in the UK – a job I loved – and came here, to Hanoi. Two years later I am still here and am putting the final touches to my first book. When I'm not writing, I am teaching English.

Managing my sugar levels here is also a new challenge for me. In my first few months it was difficult. My diet had completely changed. I was finding myself needing less and less insulin as I got used to what is actually a much healthier diet for me. Of course Vietnam is famous for producing rice. And I consume my fair share the odd lunch time. But in general I eat a very low GI, vegetable based diet that has been great for my sugar level control. Eating out on the street, as I do most days, is difficult because I never know exactly what is being put in to each dish. But I have slowly begun to figure it out - as we do with everything new.

Who knows whether or not I would have ended up here had I not been Diabetic. I think my Diabetes is often a motivation for me to push myself to do the stuff I dream of doing. Just so I can prove to myself that I can do it. There are lots and lots of Type 1 Diabetics out there who have done amazing things in their lives, including those elite sportspeople who really are an inspiration to me. They are real-life examples of the things you can achieve whilst managing your Diabetes.

So there it is. Hopefully I have told you something interesting. Manage your Diabetes as best you can whilst going out and living your life – however you want to live it. Test your sugar levels five times a day. Eat low GI foods. Make sure people know about your condition. Do all the stuff I've written in the past thirteen chapters. And share your experience. There are newly diagnosed Type 1 Diabetics around the world every day. As time passes and you become the expert of your own condition, pass your knowledge on to help others. I'll be out there looking for your tips.

Disclaimer

This book is not intended as a substitute for the medical advice of physicians. The reader should regularly consult a physician in matters relating to his/her health and particularly with respect to any symptoms that may require diagnosis or medical attention.

In other words, the advice I have offered in this book is based on my own experience of Type 1 Diabetes and is my own opinion. I do not claim to be an expert or a doctor.

The book should be read, and my advice considered, in conjunction with regular visits to the professionals.

Printed in Great Britain
by Amazon